A Life Unburdened

Getting Over Weight and Getting On With My Life

Richard Morris

MIRALIBRI PRESS

Wonderful Books and Media

contact@miralibripress.com

C O P Y R I G H T

Published by Miralibri Press
P.O. Box 2452 Woodbridge, VA 22195
contact@miralibripress.com

First Printing, November 2005

Printed in the United States of America

Library of Congress Control Number: 2005933912

ISBN 0-9772842-0-4

Publisher's Note: This book is not intended as a substitute for medical advice. The
contents are provided with the aim of sharing the personal experiences and opinions of
the author for informational purposes only. Neither the publisher nor the author shall
be held liable for any consequences resulting or allegedly resulting from any action
undertaken by any person reading, or following the information in this book.
Consequently, neither the publisher nor the author is responsible for any condition you
have, or may have in the future, that may require medical supervision. Additionally, you
are advised and encouraged to confer with your health care provider regarding the
undertaking of any actions or the existence of any medical conditions that affect your
health.

Internet addresses, book titles, and author information were accurate up to the date of
publication. Neither the publisher nor the author shall be held liable for any errors or
changes that occur after the date of publication.

DEDICATION

To my wife Mary,
and my daughters, Stephanie and Raven

To Beth,

In good health.

Mary L. Morris

ACKNOWLEDGMENTS

In *Think And Grow Rich*, motivational writer Napoleon Hill introduces readers to the Master Mind Principle, which states that when two or more people come together, to apply their intellects toward a common goal, great things can happen. This book is a testament to the power of the Master Mind, and to the enduring faith of like-minded friends, family, and associates. You can never say thank you enough to the people who help you reach your goals, but you should always try.

I would like to acknowledge the nucleus of my Master Mind by saying thank you to my wife Mary, and to my daughters, Stephanie and Raven. There were several key people who provided their professional expertise and personal time to this project and made it better. They are Carol Morris, Teri Miller, Alana Sugar, C.N., Sharon Wong, Katherine Czapp and Sally Fallon.

I must also accord special recognition to the Weston A. Price Foundation, its enthusiastic members, and all the dedicated farmers and independent producers who work hard every day to provide families with real information, and real food, the right way.

Thank you all for your assistance, your energy, and your encouragement. Finally, to Cora Morris, as always, you were right. Thank you.

TABLE OF CONTENTS

Foreword

A Life Unburdened
by Sally Fallon

What happens when a fat man who should have been a stand-up comic loses over 160 pounds and then writes about it? You get a book that is funny, sad, insightful, interesting, readable and inspirational.

What happens when a fat man who's failed at all the diets stops blaming his lack of willpower and figures out that all the expert advice on dieting is wrong? You get a truly practical road map to successful weight loss.

What happens when a fat man wakes up to the fact that the only way to achieve real health is to eat real food? You get stunning, inspiring life-style transformation.

A Life Unburdened is a myth-breaker. Richard Morris demolishes them one after another: the myth that eating fat makes you fat, the myth that no food is better than any other food, the myth that junk food in moderation won't hurt you, the myth that all calories are the same, the myth that no one has time to cook, the myth that losing weight will automatically make you healthy, the myth that exercise will cure disease. Morris sheds myths the way he has shed pounds, emerging as a new man from the fog of misinformation.

His program is simple. . . and absolutely radical: don't eat processed food. Ever. Eat only real food and only when you have prepared it yourself.

And what is real food? All the foods the experts have told us not to eat: butter, lard, beef, whole raw milk, eggs, liver, coconut, cream.

His message is absolutely liberating: the only way to lose weight and be healthy is to eat foods that are satisfying. Satisfying foods are foods that contain the F word—fat, old-fashioned fats, which our ancestors ate. Satisfying foods are foods prepared the way your grandmother made them, with soupbones and love. Satisfying foods are foods that give your body what it needs, so you're not hungry an hour later. Satisfying foods grow in gardens nearby, not monocropped furrows in far-off places. Satisfying foods come from animals that live outdoors, not in factories. Satisfying foods have not been adulterated, embalmed, emulsified, sterilized, pasteurized, irradiated, manipulated or standardized.

Morris arrives at his breathtaking epiphany by asking the right questions. Why were the members of his family getting fatter, and fatter sooner, with each generation? Why were they dying so young? Why did he keep hearing that food should be convenient? Why did dieting make him depressed and lethargic? Why did the "experts," the MDs, PhDs and RDs, keep promoting the same dietary advice when it obviously was not working?

Morris does not have a bunch of letters after his name but he has a different kind of credentials—he's been there, been in the trenches. He has lived the physical and emotional agony of being fat. He has lost weight on all the diets—before gaining it all back and more. And he has achieved the supreme accomplishment of transforming himself from an obese to a normal man by making one revolutionary change: real food instead of processed food. Everything else followed from there— slow and steady weight loss, a rebirth of optimism, the end of cravings, resolution of health problems, enthusiasm for exercise, new goals, improved family life, hope for the future.

Foreword

. . . .

A Life Unburdened is more than just a diet book, it is a saga, and more than a saga of one man only, but of a couple and a family, a saga in which the discerning and supportive role of Richard's wife Mary emerges as an example of quiet heroics. It is a modern epic of self-transformation, one that unfolds with suspense and drama, as one suburban family replaces commercialism with wise principles. It begins in despair and ends in triumph.

Read, learn and enjoy!

Sally Fallon, President
The Weston A. Price Foundation
October, 2005

Part One
A Personal Journey

Introduction

Is today the day I die?

Is today the day I die?

This is the wrong question for a 43-year-old to ask himself, but there it was again, the question that had become as much a part of my life as the symphony of pain that greeted me every morning. The persistent nightmares of drowning that left me breathless in the dark hours, and the mad drumming of my heart at the slightest exertion during the day kept the specter of death on my mind constantly.

The sole source of my despair was my declining health. My life was a pond into which obesity and poor health had come crashing like a stone. The resulting ripple affected everything: my career, my family and my own self image. I feared I would not live long enough to see my children reach adulthood.

In the book of John, chapters 11 and 12, we learn of Lazarus, brother of Mary and Martha of Bethany. Lazarus was well acquainted with death, having spent four days in the tomb until he miraculously rose from the grave at the spoken word of Jesus. Weighing in at over 400 pounds on my six-foot frame, I felt as though I were already dead, a walking sarcophagus, my life entombed in my own body. Who would rescue me?

I was not alone. According to the Centers for Disease Control, up to two-thirds of Americans are either overweight or obese, and are at an increased risk of weight-related illness. The clinical definitions of overweight and obesity are different, based on the "body mass index" or BMI. BMI is a height-weight standard sanctioned by the government. Overweight is defined as having a BMI greater than 25, while a BMI greater than 30 is defined as obese. Anything above 40 is considered morbidly obese. There is some disagreement among experts regarding where exactly, the thresholds for these weight categories should fall. For the sake of simplicity, except where noted, I will use the terms overweight and obese interchangeably to refer to a physical state that is above a healthy weight for an individual.

These days, it's easy to find plenty of alarming news about America's expanding waistline, and the associated health problems that come with it. The newspapers, television and the internet are full of sobering stories about obesity-related diseases, miracle diet drugs and a never-ending stream of "fast" and "easy" weight loss solutions. For years diet experts have been telling us how to lose weight, but somehow their advice just doesn't seem to work for most of us. Even when we do manage to lose some weight, even after all the dieting, deprivation and depression, we gain it all back. We've been told that our failure is proof of our personal weakness and evidence of a masochistic desire to be fat. Many of us have accepted this explanation, even though deep down we know it isn't true.

The health problems that become part of your life once excessive weight reaches a critical level are too numerous to mention here, but there is one problem that I must address now, in order that you may understand how my wife and I eventually found success. This problem is the rift between the tidy conclusions of weight-loss science as understood by many professionals, and the messy truth of weight-gain reality that people face every day.

Over the last fifteen years, as I graduated from overweight to obese to morbidly obese, I had the sense that no one really understood what I was going through. This was especially true of the medical professionals whose advice to "push away from the table," "eat in moderation" and "get plenty of exercise" had absolutely no connection to the real world I lived in. I couldn't push away from the table because I didn't know when I'd had enough. Eating in moderation sounded like a fine idea, but no one could explain to me how to do it without needing to binge later on. And how could I get plenty of exercise when standing for more than five minutes was exhausting? Even today, despite the unprecedented attention given to the matter of obesity, the disconnect between what the professionals believe and what many overweight people experience still exists.

I believe this problem is directly linked to the fact that many of the professionals who treat patients with weight-related health problems have little first hand knowledge of the challenges these people face. The problem is compounded when obesity is seen not as a health problem, but as a moral failing. Even the concept of overeating, when generically applied to anyone who is overweight, can contribute to this disconnect, because sometimes what appears to be a problem of overeating is really a problem of undernourishment. One of the quirks of human behavior is our natural inclination to assume others see and experience life as we do. The oft repeated phrase, "If I can do it, you can too," directed at an overweight person who clearly can't "do it," at least not in the way the speaker is suggesting, is evidence of this perceptual flaw in human behavior. There is, of course, some truth in the basic premise that people can modify their behavior and change their life. It's what this book is about after all, but unless a health professional has walked in the shoes of his clients, is exceptionally empathetic or is highly skilled in the nutrition and behavioral sciences, he may never really be able to reach those people in a manner that is meaningful.

Some things are so personal and so painful that a person suffering from obesity may not be able to tell them to their doctor. Likewise, some beliefs about nutrition and health are so deeply embedded in our behavior that we may not know *ourselves* why we eat and behave the way we do. How can doctors, many of whom lack sufficient training in nutrition, be of any use beyond writing prescriptions for the treatment of disorders associated with excess weight? This becomes a typical scenario when, despite their best efforts, many doctors must become misers with their time in order to service a growing patient load. Byzantine insurance plans, pharmaceutical industry influence, increased patient costs and declining levels of service have steadily chipped away at the doctor-patient relationship until doctors rarely even speak to their patients anymore.

I do not mean to imply that the medical community is of no use in this regard. To the contrary, much of the useful advice about nutrition, weight loss and health that can be acquired today comes as a result of the efforts of some very fine physicians, scientists and researchers, past and present. But there is another element, another voice that is conspicuously absent from the national dialog that drives policy on obesity and lifestyle recommendations. This voice cannot be found in the lofty towers of scientific conformity. Very often, it cannot be found between the covers of most weight-loss books written by experts with "years of clinical experience dealing with overweight patients." To hear this voice, you must listen to someone who's been there, in the trenches and minefields, and in the kitchens and convenience stores, of Main Street, America, where the real battle for personal health is fought.

This book, then, is not an account of a carefully controlled double-blind placebo study conducted with overweight, nonsmoking, left handed men with a median age of 35. Nor does it present theory and conjecture based on a meta-analysis of raw data extrapolated from long-term studies involving obese lab rats. What this book is about is a real American family in the real world, faced with the very real challenge of what to do about our declining health. It is about how we leveraged the knowledge of the information age and applied it, in this, the new age of self determination. It is about how we overcame obesity, clinical depression and a host of other illnesses by applying a ten-step methodology. And it's about how we closed the gap between theoretical nutrition science and the everyday reality of two-for-one hamburgers, and how you can do the same.

. . . .

THE LAZARUS PROJECT

"I want my life back." Those were the words, spoken to my wife Mary, on a forgotten day in a year long faded from memory. In those words, I expressed the deepest sorrow of a life once flush with the bloom of human potential.

In June of 2003, Mary and I decided it was time to take responsibility for our health. We vowed to learn everything we could about nutrition and health and apply it to our lives. At the time, we felt as though we were the walking dead, and longed for the day when we could live again. We weren't just doing this for ourselves, either. The health of our two daughters was at stake as well. It seemed a fitting name to call our experiment the Lazarus Project. Eighteen months later, we found ourselves, like Lazarus, risen from the metaphorical grave of a life weighted down with obesity and disease. We found that as our physical problems diminished, we quite literally grew younger in both mind and body. In no time, we found that we had more energy than we could handle. Suddenly our world seemed full of promise, and we began to realize that it really was possible to create happiness in our lives. Whether that happiness comes in the form of an improved relationship with someone you love, a better career, or the courage to pursue your dreams, it can all be yours for the taking. What was at the center of this wonderful and dramatic change we experienced? Food!

Some health professionals tell us that it doesn't matter what we eat so long as we watch the calories. They tell us that all food is the same and that it is quantity, not quality, that is important when it comes to managing our weight and our health. We have discovered that this is simply not true. It is a lie that has condemned several members of our own family, and countless others, to a life of illness and an early grave. We discovered that food really does matter, more than we imagined. This simple "secret" is the foundation upon which we designed our own resurrection from illness and our escape from a life of despair.

The first section of this book, "A Personal Journey," looks back at where we were, beginning with a painfully detailed journal of what it was like for my wife and myself to deal with obesity and the associated health problems on a daily basis. Later, in the chapter "Dieting in the Dark," we revisit some of the diets we've tried over the years in a stroll down dieting memory lane.

The second section, "Losing Our Way," talks about the evolution of the food industry, the transition from home-cooked meals to processed convenience foods, and takes a behind-the-scenes look at how industry influences what we eat and ultimately how healthy we are. The third section, "The Road Home," details what we learned, and what we did to get over weight and get on with our lives. In the fourth section, "It's All About the Food," you'll get an insider's view of what's in my pantry and learn how to use the Total Food Index, a powerful tool to help you make better decisions about what you eat. Finally, the last section, "Rebirth," shares the story of a difficult challenge we faced to test both our bodies and our spirits. In this section, we reveal the ten-step methodology we applied to change our lives forever.

Like Lazarus, we discovered that after death comes life. We want to share some of what we've learned and start you on your own journey toward getting over weight and getting on with a new life of better health and the discovery of your own greater potential.

Chapter One

A Day in the Life
Of a Fat Man
Twenty-four hours, 400 pounds and 1 Big Apple

I've read that people who lose a leg or an arm can sometimes feel a phantom pain in the missing limb. I had all of my parts thankfully, but there it was again, the faint memory of a crippling leg cramp from almost two decades ago. I remembered the pain, the extreme fatigue, and worst of all, the memory loss and a nearly complete blackout.

Standing on the south rim of the Grand Canyon with my wife, Mary, the memories came back, even as I took in the wonder of the canyon. A sea of fantastic rock formations in brilliant hues of amber and crimson rolled to the distant horizon like an ocean of petrified waves beneath the gathering clouds of an approaching storm. My eyes followed a mule train as it wound its way up the steep and twisting trail out of the depths of the abyss. The trail plunged more than 3000 feet to the edge of a plateau that lay in the hazy distance a little more than six miles off. Six miles, a short distance relatively speaking, but six miles down and six miles back, into and out of the canyon, represented a level of difficulty that was an order of magnitude greater than the pleasant strolls we enjoyed back home, along the paved and gently rolling hills of suburban Virginia.

The last time we made this trip was 1986, 18 years ago. I was three years out of college and just 26 years old at the time. Newly married, I was ready to take on the world. Although I had already started to put on weight, I still had the physique of one accustomed to strenuous exercise. In those days, I could run for miles, cared little about what I ate, and felt as though I just might live forever. I had no idea what a tragic turn my health would take over the coming decades.

By May of 2003, I was a dead man walking. At more than 400 pounds, I suffered from a constellation of obesity-related ills that included shortness of breath, sleep apnea, hypertension, aches and pains in my joints, depression, a frail immune system and a checklist of other ailments too numerous to list here. Simply standing was painful and walking, even on flat turf, was exhausting beyond a short distance. Every part of my body complained of one ache or another. Bloated and ill, I had become an old man long before my time, and was haunted daily by the specter of an untimely death. I had long since mothballed dreams of hiking the canyon again.

And yet here I stood in February, 2005, less than two years later, completely reborn and ready to take on one of the most challenging day hikes found anywhere in the lower forty-eight states. At 250 pounds, I was still a big man by most estimates, but the body that once carried over 160 pounds of excess fat now sported an astonishingly slimmer physique and hardened muscle. This transformation left me with an unshakable faith that given the right motivation, we really can move mountains. My new life owed much to a year's worth of newly acquired knowledge about nutrition. During the period of weight loss—all 160 pounds of it—I enjoyed some of the most delicious meals of my life. I also discovered that regular exercise isn't supposed to hurt and that the post-workout pain I suffered in college was really an early indication of a poor diet and my declining health.

Mary experienced a similar transformation, shedding fifty pounds while regaining her youthful figure and zest for life. Tomorrow we would be heading down the south rim's Bright Angel trail for the first time in 18 years. We had been preparing for this challenge for well over a year, but were we ready? Would we make it? Winter in the canyon is no joke, and there was snow in the forecast for tomorrow. The question, "Would we make it?" kept repeating in my mind. As I stood there and looked out over the unforgiving landscape, I felt like an explorer about to embark on a journey into a harsh and uncompromising world. I have been to such a place before, trapped in my old life as a fat man. If you've never been there yourself, let me give you some idea of what it was like.

A DIFFERENT WORLD

What does it feel like to be really fat? If you've never been there, it may be difficult to comprehend. There are a complex series of factors, both physical and emotional, that combine to create an experience quite unlike anything else. You might say that the reality of being fat is so unlike anything else that fat people live in an entirely different world.

Theirs is a world where the pull of gravity exerts a greater-than-normal toll on the body. The sun is hotter, even in winter, and the air is always thinner. In a twist of bitter irony, everything is smaller in this world, everything that is, except the people: cars, bathrooms, restaurant booths, even clothing seem designed to create the maximum amount of discomfort.

The chief preoccupation for the inhabitants of this world is the never-ending search for contentment. It is a search forever thwarted by an unfulfilled hunger and an unquenchable thirst. Self control is nonexistent in this part of the galaxy.

This world is littered with the corpses of failed dreams and missed opportunities. Humor comes at the price of personal dignity. Self doubt and insecurity are constant companions, as are pain, illness and the ever-present shadow of premature death. Only the stout of heart and body can survive here, but no one really survives for very long. When death comes, for many, it comes not a moment too soon.

6:00am Tuesday

The buzzing in my head is the perfect accompaniment to the dull pain that throbs just behind my temples. The two sensations fuse to create an image of a large mechanical insect with a long, syringe-like stinger, drilling deep into my skull. The buzzing comes from my tormentor, a small alarm clock perched on the bedside table just beyond my reach. Like a lot of things recently, it is a new and unwelcome addition to my life. The pain in my head is quite a different matter. For the past month or so, it has visited me nearly every morning. I can't say whether it's the stress in my life or the high blood pressure that is causing the headaches, but I've grown quite accustomed to them. I lash out at the alarm clock, my arms flailing until, by accident more than aptitude, I hit the snooze button.

As I lie quietly in the half-dark of my room, a thin film of sweat settles over me in the still humid air. I try to drift off to sleep again, but my circadian clock is no less aware of the time than the clock on the table. I began to notice other sounds now: the steady hum of the ice machine down the hall, and the beating of my own heart. Last night had been a blessing. Though I had not slept well, I had slept long enough to achieve something remotely similar to a night's rest. Still, the knot of tension in my neck had not abated; worse, it had spread tendrils through my shoulders and down into my back. The ritual sadism of daylight savings time, too-rich hotel food, and the stress of working in the gulag that is my job, has sucked the life from me. I am a corpse on a slab, bloated and ripe for dissection.

My brain feels like an old computer running on an outdated operating system. It's not uncommon, as I transition from the unconscious world to the waking world, to experience a moment of confusion before all of the details of my life are properly loaded into my short term memory. Like a pilot preparing for takeoff, I run through my own personal checklist. I am in a hotel room in New York City, lower Manhattan to be exact. Check. I am on the 10th—no, that was last week— the 20th floor of a downtown hotel. Check. I am on a temporary assignment to work on a large software development project. Check. Temporary is a relative term, as it has been well over four months since I began making the three hour Monday morning slog up the northeast corridor from my home in Virginia. Today is Tuesday, the morning of our weekly project status meeting. My heart sinks at the very thought of it. I wish I were someplace, anyplace, other than here. Double check.

I lie in bed on my back, feeling just as tired and used up as I had when I lay down the night before. Morning light begins filtering past the thin veil of my eyelids, forcing me to squint. An inner voice whispers faintly in my ear with the subtle and subtlety of a serpent's tongue, "Another day in the factory." Just then, the clock starts up again with its incessant buzzing. Get up, get up! I roll onto my side and reach for it; then, with much effort, sit up and pivot to the edge of the bed. I slump here for a moment and wait for the room to stop spinning and the headache to subside. It takes effort to do a lot of things these days. The aches and pains that accompany the day's first stirrings are a familiar morning ritual for many, but for me, a middle-aged man of 43 years, beset with asthma, high blood pressure and an astonishing body weight, it is just the beginning of another twenty-four hours of humiliation and misery.

Amid grunts and audible popping sounds coming from my joints, I rise from the bed and stumble past the clothes strewn about the floor to the window. An explosion of aches and pains ricochets through my body from my ears to my ankles and back again. I feel like I've been hit with a blast of buckshot from point-blank range, and yet, I am so accustomed to feeling this way that I hardly notice it anymore. My only concern on this late spring morning, as it has been every morning recently, is just figuring out how I will make it through another day. I part the curtains and squint into the full light of a New York morning. I'm facing south, just north of Battery Park. The view of the Hudson River is obscured by an apartment building directly in front of me. To the left, a fortress of buildings obliterates the horizon. Here and there, I can see morning ferries and tug boats crisscrossing the slate grey waters of the Hudson, and beyond that, a swath of the Jersey shore. Twenty floors down, West Street bustles with early morning traffic.

I have what some might call a dream job: a high profile position on a major corporate project, company paid expenses, and one of the greatest cities in the world at my feet. And yet, I can't get past the simple fact that I'm not enjoying any of it. Certainly my weight is a factor, but is it the primary factor? Before writing this book, I would have been unsure of the answer to that question, but I now know that the 200 extra pounds I carried with me everyday were like a thick, nearly opaque lens, through which every thought and every experience of my life was filtered.

As I stand here, I wonder what Mary and the girls are doing back home in Virginia. At 6:00 in the morning, they're probably still asleep. The separation has been difficult for all of us. I should feel good, after all, as I was fulfilling the chief tenet of manhood, which is to care for one's family. As the sole breadwinner, I was doing just that. In fact, I took a certain masochistic pride in the fact that through it all, I was still holding up. But this was just testosterone-induced bravado. The fact is, I felt as if I was letting them down. By my own estimation, I had fallen far short of the goals I had set for myself as a husband and father.

My relationship with Mary suffered because, when I got right down to it, I didn't really like who I was. My weight and the associated health problems made me feel weak and a failure; it's hard to give love when you don't have any to spare for yourself. Mary had her own problems. A 50-pound surplus of body weight and an even deeper emotional scar that had plagued her since childhood made us like two speeding cars on a collision trajectory, our combined problems magnifying the force of impact. Worse still, I perceived that our joint failure at setting a good example was priming our daughters for a lifetime of unnecessary pain and suffering.

I shower and dress quickly. I always do, because being fat means that your wardrobe will be severely limited, making the decision of what to wear most mornings a no-brainer. I pull on a pair of dark pants, and tuck in a white dress shirt. A lightweight tan sweater goes over the shirt. I choose the sweater even though the weather is warming up. When you're my size, sweaters tend to soften the contrast between the mound of belly fat and your lower body. On this day, I will wear a heavy leather coat over my sweater, as the evenings in New York are still quite cool.

I look in the mirror and unconsciously sneer at the man who returns my stare. My face is puffed and swollen, with the beginnings of dark circles forming around my eyes to complement the darkening splotches on my cheeks. At six feet tall, I am above average height, but the overall effect is ruined by the rolling mounds of flesh that pour down from my chest ending abruptly in a great orbital ring of fat around my midsection. The once youthful shimmer of my skin is gone, replaced with a flat and ashen mask, reminding me of the last glimpse of my father as he lay in his coffin.

Between my waist and my neck, I'm almost round. My clothes always fit poorly. Sometimes they are too large while at other times too small. I am always out of fashion. This isn't because of a lack of availability of stylish clothing. The fashion industry caters rather well to the ever-expanding waistline of the American male, but given the exorbitant prices for big-sized clothing, almost a penalty for being overweight, many simply cannot afford to buy better clothes.

I can feel swelling in my hands. My feet, with their poor circulation and blackened toenails, thankfully hidden in my shoes, look like something from a grade-B horror movie. The specter of diabetes that has shadowed three members of my immediate family haunts me daily.

The tired, dull eyes that stare back at me are hardly recognizable as my own. Somehow I have still managed to retain a memory of what I used to look like. I do not recognize this man in the mirror.

The circumference of my waist, being nearly equal to my height, requires me to wear my pants farther down, around my hips. I never liked wearing suspenders as hitching my pants high up on the waist makes me look too much like the Pentecostal preachers that shepherded the churches of my youth. When I do wear a belt, the weight of my overhanging stomach rubs against the belt buckle creating a painful abrasion that sometimes breaks the skin and bleeds. Some days it is so painful I have to go to the restroom at work and stuff a wad of tissue paper between my stomach and the belt buckle.

It occurs to me that life with obesity is much like my belt, an ever-tightening noose that is slowly cutting me off from everything and everyone I know. Some days are worse than others, but these days, it seems there are no more good days left. As bad as this morning is, it is about to get worse.

7:30am

I go down to the hotel restaurant for breakfast. I am usually still full from my evening meal and often skip breakfast, but being full and being satiated are two different things. I order from the buffet menu and have an omelet, grits (I was amazed to find grits in New York City), orange juice and sausage. Eating in public carries with it a special risk and countless opportunities for humiliation. I try to ignore the stares, the sidelong glances, and the way some people's eyes dart briefly to take in my stomach before reestablishing eye contact. The hostess is a young attractive woman who is all smiles and kind words, but I know or think I know what she and everyone else in the restaurant is thinking: look at that fat guy stuff himself with fried eggs and sausage.

8:00am

The walk to the office is difficult. It's only a few blocks, but it feels like miles to me, even though it's mostly downhill. I know I'll have to come back this way in the evening, and do not look forward to it. New Yorkers have seen it all, so I'm almost relieved to discover that I don't draw as many stares as I normally do. I don't see many children on the street in lower Manhattan during morning rush, but on this day a mother and child of about five years rush by. The kid is wailing for something, but stops mid-wail to gawk at me. Mom glances at me for a moment then pulls him forward and the wail picks up again. I imagine he's probably begging for sweets and can hear, if only in my mind, the mother warning him that if he eats too much candy, "you'll wind up like that fat man."

One: A Day in the Life Of a Fat Man

. . . .

Even though it is cool in the mornings, my size and poor condition cause my internal furnace to heat up quickly. By the time I get to my building several blocks away, I'm almost out of breath. I nod to the security guard as I make my way to the elevators. The lobby is nearly empty. As I step onto the elevator, my mind is preoccupied with the coming events of the day, so I am unprepared for what happens next.

One moment I'm in mid-stride with one leg raised above the threshold of the elevator. The next, when my foot comes down and touches the elevator floor, my left knee gives out. For an instant, I'm in danger of crashing to the floor, but I catch myself and stumble against the wall. This isn't the first time this has happened, but I note with a sense of disquiet that it is happening with greater frequency. Joint and mobility problems are common complaints of the morbidly obese. I wonder how long will it be before I can no longer walk without aid?

I finally make it up to my floor where I collapse at my desk. I'm sweating profusely and breathing heavily. I wipe the sweat from my brow, but like a garden sprinkler, more pours out of me. The white shirt beneath the sweater I'm wearing is soaked through. It takes several minutes for my breathing and my racing heart to return to normal. It will take twenty minutes or more for my shirt to dry out. For those people who say the obese need to "just get out and exercise," I have this to say: Try walking in my shoes for a day.

9:00am

I work as a software design liaison between my company and an outside contractor. I spend most of my day sitting in meetings or at a desk. This is the blessing and the curse of modern technology, which gives us the miracle of enhanced productivity through the use of computers, while exacting a heavy toll on our health.

Like the animals on a modern day factory farm, I feel trapped and unable to direct the course of my own future. The vending machine down the hall spits out soda for twenty-five cents a can—such a deal. High-calorie, low-nutrient donuts, bagels, pizza, and other goodies are regularly supplied by my employer, at little or no cost. My coworkers and I often eat hurriedly at our desks, barely tasting the food. We are like beef on the hoof, fattened up on a high-grain diet, and crowded into a feed lot awaiting slaughter at the whim of our corporate masters. Sometimes when I close my eyes, I can almost hear mooing.

The hours are often long, and due to the complexity of the work, problems, or should I say, "challenges," the politically correct corporate euphemism, are legion. Along with these challenges comes a super sized helping of stress. I was about to get my first serving at our morning meeting. The room in which the meeting is held is ridiculously small for the number of people attending. I get there early so I can pick a seat at the table that's easy to get to and doesn't require others to squeeze past me. Other people begin streaming into the room. Everyone looks as if they've enjoyed a better night's rest than I did. While almost everyone else looks crisp and freshly attired, I look worn and feel worse and the day has only just begun. I try to keep up with the dialog, but find that I'm having a difficult time concentrating. This is a growing and more frequent problem. When it is my turn to report, I stumble through my script in a lifeless monotone, not sure if I'm making any sense, and hoping no one asks any questions.

10:00am

An unexpected meeting comes up that is located in another building a couple of blocks away. This is bad news because it means that not only will I have to go walking, but I won't be alone. When I'm walking by myself, I can walk at my own pace, stopping now and then to rest, but I know I'll have to keep pace with the energetic young man who will accompany me to the meeting. We start out along Broad Street and head toward the end of the block, not far from the stock exchange. A left turn takes us up a long incline toward Broadway. My heart is pounding. Pride prevents me from admitting that I need to rest. The leather coat makes me feel like I'm wearing a portable sauna, and my breathing is barely under control. Talking is difficult. By the time we arrive at the meeting, I am drenched and exhausted. For the next ten minutes, so much sweat pours from my head and face that I must look like a fountain in a park. I certainly feel as though I weigh as much. The only thing missing, I muse, is the pigeons.

12:00pm

There are problems—there always are—with the project. Another unscheduled meeting comes up. I've barely returned from my last appointment when I have to go out again, this time for a lunch meeting with one of the project's principal clients as well as a group of managers from my company. The restaurant is close by, but small. I find that I have difficulty negotiating the narrow passages between tables to get to my seat. The shirt beneath my sweater is still damp and as I sit there, I can sense that a few buttons have come undone and that my shirttail has crept up out of my pants.

One of the problems with being obese is that when you sit at a table, your stomach forces you to sit much farther away from the table than normal. Food has to travel a greater distance from the plate to your mouth. Spills occur often. I'm careful to order the salmon as it is relatively easy to control, unlike spaghetti or a salad, which would have been a disaster. I thank God that at least we're at a table and not a booth. Booths are unequaled in the depth of physical discomfort and public humiliation they offer to the obese. They are the modern-day equivalent of a medieval "iron lady," designed to force fat people to choose between talking and breathing.

Just as I was beginning to settle into the conversation and momentarily forget about my personal troubles, disaster strikes. Because I jut so far out into the aisle, one of the waiters, balancing a tray of coffee cups and cream, bumps into me and spills cream all over my back. I can feel the cold, viscous liquid creeping down my shirt. The waiter grabs a towel and between apologies begins sopping up the cream as best he can. He implores me to remove my sweater so that he can have it cleaned at the restaurant's expense.

Everyone at my table and the tables around me is staring. I am now faced with a difficult choice: remove my sweater and reveal my sweat-stained, ill-fitting, partially unbuttoned shirt and the mounds beneath, or refuse the offer to have my sweater cleaned and look like the village idiot in front of the entire restaurant. I choose to be an idiot and lamely try to laugh off the incident, declining the waiter's offer.

I think this scene can't get any worse, but I am wrong. Now the restaurant manager, a young attractive woman, comes over and again insists that I remove my sweater so the restaurant can have it cleaned. It isn't often that strange women demand I undress in public, so I find I'm at a loss for words. I tell her I'm from out of town and she counters that she'll have the sweater sent to wherever I live. The restaurant is nearly dead silent as I struggle for a response.

"No it's OK, really," I mutter.

My table-mates are looking at me now as though I really am from another world. It feels like ages before the hum of normal conversation picks up again and people return to their business. Whatever opinion my coworkers at the table had of me when we entered the restaurant, I'm now certain it is markedly different when we leave. In a final stab of humiliation, as we're leaving the restaurant, the manager asks me once more whether I would like to have my sweater cleaned. I thank her and reply that I'm staying just a few blocks away and will go change clothes after lunch. To add a final insult to my injury, I tip the coat girl far more than she deserves. No one mentions the incident on the walk back to the office. I step across a large metal grate in the street through which the sound and the fury of a passing subway train can be heard and almost wish the grate would give way and swallow me up.

2:00pm

I spend the rest of the day hiding at my desk. I need a shower and feel sticky in clothes that have been twice dampened by sweat, and now by cream. It's starting to rain outside.

Usually at about this time, I get drowsy and nod off. I try to stay awake by keeping busy making phone calls and attacking my to-do list. These episodes of midday sleepiness usually pass in about an hour.

3:00pm

Another meeting. I have a phone call and arrive late. There's no place to sit, so I stand. My lower back is killing me. Someone leaves early and I grab his chair. Halfway into it, I discover that it's too small for me. I'm wedged between the armrests. If I try to stand up, the chair will come with me, so I squeeze into it. Everyone pretends not to notice my predicament.

4:00pm

Andy, one of the guys in the office, invites me to come along to dinner with a group of programmers. I pretend to consider the offer before declining. I've learned that a dinner invitation means strolling aimlessly for blocks until the group discovers a restaurant that looks interesting. The last time I accepted a dinner invitation, the exhausting walk to the restaurant killed my appetite while the walk back, as difficult as it was on a full stomach, only made me hungry shortly after I returned to my room.

Every day I vow to accept the dinner invitations from the New York staff and accompany them to one of the many restaurants in the area. Every night I find another reason not to. The reasons typically fall into one of three categories: work, family or illness. Tonight was "illness" night. I said that I must be coming down with something and needed to get to bed early. Andy smiles and says something about "the next time then."

There's always a next time when you're obese. The next diet will be the one that works for me, or next week I'm really going to try harder to exercise more. We spend most of our working day in hopeful yet hopeless anticipation of the next this, the next that, that never comes.

By the end of the day, I'm drenched and exhausted. At least today, I'll actually get to leave at a respectable hour. On some days, people are here all night. The glamorous world of software development isn't so glamorous after all, I muse.

WHAT GOES AROUND, COMES AROUND
5:00pm

Rain has been falling in a light, steady drizzle ever since the early afternoon, creating puddles everywhere of grimy blackish soup. The evening rush of foot traffic pours out of the buildings and surges into the street, a gray wave of humanity. People walk with heads down, eyes forward, swirling around and past me as though I am a large stone in the midst of a great silent river. I lumber up a long wide alleyway that inclines toward Broadway. The hotel is still several blocks away, but it feels like I've already walked several miles. The trauma of walking uphill after an endless day of sitting in meetings intensifies the grinding pain in my lower back. It grows worse with each step. I can feel the eyes of the crowd all around me, can feel the suffocating waves of pity and disgust that threaten to drown me.

As I step off a curb, my foot sinks into a puddle of water. After months of walking through dirty snow and water, my shoes are ruined and now they are soaked through to the socks. I heave myself forward, dodging a cab before reaching the relative safety of the opposite curb.

5:20pm

I sit on the edge of the bed in my small sterile room, my sweater lying crumpled behind me. Slumped and lifeless, I could pass for a large pile of dirty laundry carelessly dropped at the foot of the bed. The bedding is violently disturbed where I collapsed soon after arriving. The excruciating pain in my lower back and joints give me little choice. Some nights on the walk back to the hotel I barely make it to the privacy of the lobby elevator before collapsing in pain against the wall. I am tired inside and out.

6:00pm

Recovered from my evening walk, I decide to order dinner in my room. I almost always eat dinner in my room. The hotel restaurant is more than adequate, but after previous visits there, where the hostess seated me so far toward the back of the restaurant I could smell the dishwashing liquid in the kitchen, I took the hint. New York probably has more restaurants per square mile than any other city, but going out is just not realistic for someone like me. I shift from the bed to a tight-fitting desk chair, and absentmindedly flip through the pages of the room service menu. This is just a formality, as I have practically memorized the menu from continued use.

"Hello Mr. Morris, this is Paul. How may I help you tonight?"

The voice belongs to the Guest Services Manager. It is overtly pleasant to the point of flatness, like that of a bank officer unaccustomed to granting loan approvals. Paul and the room service staff like me. I keep them busy, tip well and am conscientious about placing the service table outside my room and phoning the desk to have someone pick it up. If the old maxim "you are what you eat," is true, Paul knows me better than he does most of the hotel's guests, as he has taken my calls many times before. Thus our familiar conversation begins.

"I'd like to order some dinner."

"Excellent Mr. Morris. Would you like to hear our special tonight?"

The line is silent for a moment. "Sure," I respond. It really doesn't matter what the special is, I've had a hard day and I need a heavy dose of comfort to put it behind me. I already know what I want.

"We start with a spicy tomato bisque soup followed by the main course, a fillet of mesquite grilled sea bass infused with truffle oils." As he works this culinary aria, the pitch and tenor of Paul's voice changes, rising in a melodic refrain that is nearly operatic. "That comes with seared asparagus spears on a bed of wild rice with fresh scallions and hand-picked mushrooms." There is a breathless pause as Paul gathers himself for the climax of this mini-opera. "For dessert, this meal includes your choice of honey-glazed baked apples in a red wine sauce or poached pears in a fragrant hibiscus-scented syrup presented in a delicate web of spun sugar."

There is the abrupt sound of a breathless exhalation as Paul cools down from the exertion. I rock back in the ill-fitting chair and wait for a moment to lend the impression that I am actually considering the special.

"Uh no, I think I'd like to go with the steak tonight."

A disappointed silence follows, then having recovered, Paul replies, "Excellent. Is that the house steak or the porterhouse?"

The house steak is a dainty 7 ounces of meat while the porterhouse weighs in at over a pound of gut-busting Colorado beef, bathed in butter and herbs.

"I'll have the porterhouse."

"How would you like that?" The color has deserted Paul's voice as he shifts back into loan officer mode.

"Medium well."

"That comes with a seafood chowder or garden salad. Which would you prefer?"

"Salad."

"Dressing?"

"Ranch. And could you put some chicken on that salad?"

"Of course. Would you like fries or mashed potatoes with your steak?"

"Fries."

"Something to drink?"

"A Coke."

"Would a Pepsi be OK?"

"Sure."

"Dessert?"

It goes like this for a moment more. The conversation is as familiar as a comfortable old chair for both of us. Like two actors with a well rehearsed script, we speak our lines with the conviction of an opening night performance. I hang up the phone and reach for the television remote, then pause and reach for the phone instead. Dinner was a half hour away. I wheel the chair around and open the in-room snack bar and smile when I see that the cache of Snickers candy bars has been replenished.

One: A Day in the Life Of a Fat Man

. . . .

6:30pm

A room service attendant brings dinner on a table tray. I sit in the ill-fitting desk chair and watch TV while I eat. Except for the prehistoric dinner rolls, which would need to be carbon dated to determine their age, the food is neither good nor bad. It simply does what all my meals do, which is to fill the hole in my belly. But never ever do my meals leave me satisfied.

8:00pm

I spend the rest of the evening sprawled uncomfortably on the bed, watching TV and flipping through the pages of a magazine. Despite the bloated feeling in my stomach and the general sense of unease that always comes after eating, I eventually attack the snack bar. In a half-hearted attempt to watch my fat intake, I skip the cookies this time and choose a can of sickeningly sweet, but stale, peanuts. They taste as though they've been languishing in a warehouse since the Reagan administration.

The willingness to eat just about anything, whether we like it or not, is one of the puzzling mysteries of the overeater. In retrospect, I realize that my insatiable cravings were the result of chronic malnourishment. This is why my meals never left me satisfied.

Before bed, I take my blood pressure medication.

2:00am

My eyes snap open. I sit up abruptly in bed, with some difficulty. I'm choking and there's a burning sensation in my throat. Acid? I cough violently trying to clear my airway. It takes a moment to remember where I am. The chunk, shush, chunk of the ice machine fills in the blanks for me. I was dreaming that I drowned.

I was unaware of it then, but dreams of drowning are not uncommon for obese people suffering from a life threatening disorder known as sleep apnea. Obstructive sleep apnea, the variant from which I suffered, is a condition whereby the airway at the back of the throat becomes periodically and temporarily blocked. The sufferer can experience frequent (as many as 60 per hour) moments of interrupted breathing. These episodes can persist throughout the night, inhibiting access to the deeper and more restful non-REM sleep stage. Snoring, daytime sleepiness and an inability to concentrate are all potential symptoms of sleep apnea. Heart attack, high blood pressure and stroke are also associated with this condition.

The pressure on my bladder cannot be ignored; disoriented, I fumble through the darkened room to the toilet. I don't trouble myself with the light switch, as my aim is no better in the light than it is in the dark. My habits have grown steadily more piggish. The longer I'm in New York, the worse I feel, the more I eat and the less I care. It is a familiar pattern that I recognize and fear, but I feel helpless to stop it. I exit the bathroom, stopping to retrieve a Pepsi from the snack bar, then step gingerly over the growing pile of clothes on the floor to the faint outline of the window across the room. Parting the curtains, I look out on a city not quite asleep.

In the pale light of a pastel moon, New York takes on the ghostly radiance of a canvas done up in translucent hues of white. In the distance, I can see the Jersey shore, loosely sketched by rows of yellow and white lights. A lone tugboat, lit up like a Christmas tree, moves silently across the water. Below me an occasional car passes, heading south, toward the West Street terminus.

6:00am Wednesday

I wake up early, squinting into the dawn light that invades the room. At some point in the night, I stumbled from my uncomfortable bed and collapsed into an uncomfortable easy chair, where I managed to sleep fitfully. The heavy meal from the previous evening leaves me dazed and feeling as though a weight greater than my own is pinning me to the chair. My mouth is parched, and thirst gnaws at me despite the evidence of several empty cans of Pepsi on the desk which I have only the faintest memory of drinking. On my first attempt to rise, my joints and unused muscles groan and protest with the effort. I fall back and contemplate what lies ahead. What goes around, comes around—another day in the Big Apple.

One: A Day in the Life Of a Fat Man

Looking back, I cannot say how I managed the burden of morbid obesity for as long I did, other than to say as my mother has said so many times before: "It was my faith that brought me." Faith can be a wonderful thing, a powerful motivator that sees us through the dark hours when our lives seem hopeless and full of bitter discontent. But faith is a double-edged sword. Applied in the wrong way, for the wrong cause, blind faith can be an anchor that pulls us down into the murky depths of self-destruction. It was blind faith that nearly destroyed me, and continues to destroy the lives of millions of people every day.

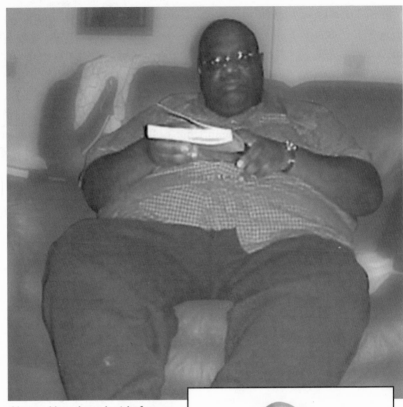

Above: Here I am just before re-locating to the East Coast. Leaving our family behind in Arizona was a tough decision, but as I said to Mary, "This move will be an opportunity for us to recreate ourselves." Little did I know how true those words were.

Right: Here I am today.

Chapter Two

How Did I End Up Here?

How a fit guy like me wound up
in a fat place like this

How did this happen? How did I wind up morbidly obese and sleepless in New York City? In high school, I lifted weights. In college, I was an avid runner, clocking four to twelve miles a day. I was also a hiker who regularly trekked into Arizona's rugged outdoors, from the Grand Canyon to the badlands of the southern desert.

I often commuted to college on my bicycle, taking on the 34-mile round trip course through rush hour traffic with the tenacity of Lance Armstrong. Once, just for kicks, I walked 17 miles home from school, under a blistering desert sun across simmering asphalt, just to prove to myself I could do it. Most people meeting me for the first time thought that I was an athlete, so how did this happen? I have asked myself this question a thousand times and only now have I begun to realize the answer. More important, after years of unsuccessful dieting, I have finally found a solution.

No one chooses to be fat. I didn't. This revelation may come as a surprise to some, but it's true. Every day we see overweight and obese people making decisions that seem to reflect a conscious choice to be fat. The lanes and parking lots at fast food restaurants are always busy with a steady flow of traffic, and we seem to be spending more time in our cars and less time walking. Snarled roads, which spread out to the distant suburbs like tentacles, keep us sitting in our cars, for hours on end, while we blindly devour fast food on our way home to eat processed convenience food that is little better. We willingly sacrifice our children to corporate America by plying them with sugary treats for breakfast, lunch and dinner. A cursory glance into the overloaded carts at your favorite big-box discount store reveals a hodgepodge of chemically enhanced, nutritionally poor convenience foods. It's easy to assume that fat people really and truly choose to be fat.

This is false logic of course, one that can easily be refuted. Most people understand quite clearly that while smokers may choose to smoke, no smoker chooses to be stricken with lung cancer. No drinker chooses to suffer the horrors of liver disease. How then do we explain the self destructive behavior of smokers, alcoholics and the obese? The mechanisms that fuel this behavior, whether an addiction, genetics, human physiology run amok or simply bad behavior are open for debate. The truth is that while many people choose to engage in injurious behavior, few will accept the consequences of that behavior.

In simple terms, smokers smoke because they enjoy the sensory experience of smoking on an emotional and physiological level. Alcoholics are little different, so too are the overweight. We all engage in behavior that gives us pleasure. The problem is that for smokers, alcoholics and overeaters, these behaviors lead to dependencies. And because of ignorance of certain truths about the food we eat, we find it all too difficult to stop. This unhealthy behavior is driven by our unmet nutritional needs and a desire for satisfaction, not by the negative consequences of the behavior.

For many people with a poor diet, immersion in this cycle of satisfaction-seeking leads to clouded judgment. Hormonal influences, which are only now being discovered, add to a scenario in which rational decision making becomes nearly impossible. So it was with me. This truth that emotional and physiological dependencies make rational behavior very difficult lies beyond the grasp of many well-intentioned health professionals who continue to focus on a simplistic, "just say no" approach to dieting.

. . . .

INDUSTRIALIZATION AND MY FAMILY

The history of America's race to industrialize the food supply is reflected in the four most recent generations of my own family. From the time my grandparents began farming over a century ago until today, amazing technological leaps have revolutionized the production, manufacture and distribution of food. The advent of food additive technology and genetically modified seeds have provided an additional and unprecedented level of control for the industries that produce our food. The rest of us, the so-called consumers, have not fared as well.

While it may appear that we have unlimited control as we choose from thousands of festively packaged items at the supermarket, that sense of control is largely an illusion. We see a range of exotic fruits and cheeses at upscale markets, but our food choices are actually more limited than we think. Lean turkeys with oversized mutated breasts dry out in the oven on Thanksgiving because we can no longer buy naturally raised turkeys with the requisite amount of body fat. We can't buy raw milk with the cream on top anymore, or beef that hasn't been raised on a diet of hormones and antibiotics. Even something as simple as finding chicken parts with the skin still on, or chicken that hasn't been soaked in "mystery broth," requires the patience of Job and the investigative powers of Sherlock Holmes.

Most of us have little idea where our food comes from, how it is produced, and how that food interacts with our bodies. Ignorance limits our ability to make the right choices about diet and nutrition since good choices can only come from good information. Artificially produced trans fats have been in our diet for decades, but our power to choose whether to consume these fats was effectively taken away by a profit motivated marketplace that failed to reveal their dangers.

The industrialization of the food supply has separated us from the origins of the food we eat, a fact reflected in the history of my family. Our story provides a cautionary tale describing how we came to lose control over our food and our lives.

FOUR GENERATIONS OF FOOD

My mother's parents were rural folk who began their lives amid the cluck and clatter of chickens, the mooing of cows, and the comforting noises of a few other barnyard residents who shared their small farm. They had a tiny patch of land in a mining camp and were little more than sharecroppers. It had been less than two-score years since the signing of the Emancipation Proclamation, but the flame of self reliance burned brightly within them and fueled their dreams for a better life than their parents had known.

Grandfather served his country as a soldier before settling down once again as a farmer and country preacher. Grandmother was an avid gardener with an extensive knowledge of the medicinal properties of the native plants that grew wild in the hills and hollows of rural Alabama.

When I was a child, my mother often recalled the work of hog killing, which usually began on a cold autumn morning. It was Grandfather's job to do the actual killing, a most solemn act. When that work was done, the hog was suspended above a wood-fired cauldron filled with boiling water drawn from the well. The animal was scalded in the water and its bristles scraped clean with a dull knife. Then the hog was slit open, disemboweled, and cut into pieces. Nothing was wasted. They made head cheese from the head, rendered lard from the skin and fat and made sausage from the innards. The pork belly and ham were salted and consigned to the smokehouse. Later, some of the lard would be used to make lye soap.

My grandparents were not rich people, and so relied mostly on the land for their subsistence. What could not be raised, hunted, caught on a hook, grown in the garden, or bartered with neighbors, was purchased from the local store. Both my mother's parents grew strong and tall, judging by the stories passed down to me and the one faded picture I have of them.

My father's parents were also farmers, resourceful and self-sufficient. Once my father took my older sister, Carol, to visit his parents on their farm in Alabama. One day, Grandmother brought in a fresh

40

batch of eggs from the henhouse and prepared to make breakfast. A city girl, Carol protested against eating "funny tasting" eggs that had been lying about the ground only a few minutes earlier. She pleaded instead for the familiar taste of commercial eggs, trussed up in a pretty carton, which she knew could be found at the local store. Our grandmother took pity on her poor misguided granddaughter and must have wondered what kind of children our father was raising. She dispatched a cousin to the store to buy eggs. Our cousin returned a short time later with store-bought eggs which Carol found more to her liking. What Carol didn't find out until much later when she was nearly grown was that those store bought eggs had actually been sold to the local grocer by my grandmother. They had come from the very same chickens. But because they had been languishing in the store for some time, they were not as fresh as the newly laid eggs grandmother had gathered for breakfast, which accounted for the difference in taste.

My own parents were born during a transitional period in the early part of the 1900s. They were less inclined to live the lives of their farming parents and sought instead to follow the bright star that lay in the northern sky and seek their fortune somewhere beyond the rural south. They lived halfway between the old world of self reliance that belonged to their parents, and the new world of dependence on automation and commercially prepared foods that was the hallmark of the new century. They settled in Detroit, and lived in a succession of houses situated on small plots of land. They kept no animals, save a few cats and a dog, but in a gesture to the lives they once knew, they regularly purchased live fowl from the farmers' market.

My father would bring a flapping, squawking chicken home on Sundays and my older brother and sister would gather round to watch him wring the bird's neck with the deft expertise of an executioner. Despite his deep longing for life in the city, he could not wring the farming spirit from his soul as easily as the life from the chicken.

The chicken was then scalded in hot water, and my brother and sister assigned to remove the feathers. My mother would gut the chicken, cut it up into as many parts as were necessary for the day's meal, and save the head, feet and other miscellaneous parts to make soup. Everything was used, save the feathers and the cluck.

Without land to call their own, my parents were rootless; they journeyed to the West Coast and back again, their lives a reflection of the restlessness of the country at large. More people were moving off the land, sometimes involuntarily, to the more transient life found in the industrial centers of urban America. Newly built highways and affordable automobiles made it impossible for anyone to stay in one place for very long. While most meals were still home-cooked, the raw ingredients for those meals came increasingly from the neighborhood store. Like most of the people of their generation, my parents consumed a greater share of these store-bought foods than their parents had and their diets included a greater percentage of refined flour and sugar. The result was the onset of excess weight and obesity in their middle years. Clearly this change was not due to a lack of exercise, as my father was a construction laborer who knew well the meaning of a hard day's work. My mother did everything from backbreaking domestic work to harvesting produce beneath a sweltering sun.

MY MOTHER'S KITCHEN

There was a time when no one in my family thought about dieting. Although some family members carried excess weight, dieting and the associated fear of food was uncommon. Food had a special meaning in our lives: more than just fuel, and more than just nourishment, food occupied a vital place in our family, as vital as our faith and our love for each other. In the turbulent 60s and even into the more tranquil 70s, the preparation and consumption of food was a fundamental part of the traditions and rituals that bound us to our family and friends.

While most of the living spaces from house to house might differ in their size and the expense of their furnishings, the kitchen was that one spot in every home that served as a common denominator. The refrigerator, stoves and sinks in the homes of my friends and extended family were all pretty much the same. The mouth-watering vision of a rib roast, the intoxicating aroma of homemade cookies, or the snap of green peas fresh from the garden were familiar sensory experiences, imbuing us all with a sense of kinsmanship.

My mother's kitchen would never have made the cover of a designer magazine, although it was the most important room in our little house with its peach colored stucco exterior and dark green trim. The house was built shotgun style, which meant you could stand at the open front door, look down the length of the house, through the kitchen and out the open back door.

The place where Momma prepared our family meals occupied a narrow space between a creaky wooden floor, covered with aging tile, and a pale green ceiling darkened with cooking smoke. It was a tunnel of delightful smells and tastes that joined our living room, in the front of the house, to an add-on room, at the rear of the house, which at one time had been a rear porch. Momma cooked on an old gas stove that was like a fire-breathing dragon. More than once, while trying to light the pilot, each of us (we were five children) had been surprised by a frightening belch of blue flame that singed our eyebrows and fanned our childish fears.

A pink Formica countertop which had a playful 1950s pattern— vaguely reminiscent of atoms—spanned the distance between the stove and the refrigerator, and held a double-sided sink of chipped porcelain. We called the refrigerator an ice-box even though none of us kids had actually ever seen a real ice-box. That term, like so many other orphaned words from my mother's generation, had yet to slumber in our collective unconscious.

Opposite the working side of the kitchen was a large horizontal freezer which, in times of plenty, we kept stocked with cuts of beef, numerous chickens, a turkey or two, pork from the squeal to the tail and fat fresh fish purchased at the grocery store or, when we were lucky, a gift fish from our neighbor, drawn from the depths of the desert lakes that lie in the northern mountains. Low-fat dieting, calorie counting, and carb-watching were not part of our lexicon or that of anyone else we knew.

A small square table with thin metal legs, shaky and insecure, stood beside the freezer. I often sat there in the evening hours, after the family meal, struggling with my homework.

My mother used heavy stainless steel pots and black-iron skillets to cook up collard greens and chili beans, scrambled eggs and country fried chicken. Soups and broths simmered patiently for hours and filled our home with delectable smells.

On cold mornings, we ate steaming bowls of oatmeal with raisins and cream, buttered grits with cheese, or flapjacks stacked three high and smothered in butter and sticky sweet, homemade syrup. Cornbread and homemade rolls awaited that first kiss of sweet butter when they came from the oven—a memory that still makes me smile from the inside out. We bought log-sized loafs of longhorn cheese from the grocer and sometimes fresh eggs from our neighbors, whose errant rooster I often pursued whenever he took a fancy to go exploring. Our milkman delivered full-fat cow's milk and goat's milk, in thick glass bottles, fresh from the dairy.

No, my mother's kitchen would never have made the cover of any designer magazine, but it will remain for me the paradigm of what a kitchen should aspire to be.

Today, our modern kitchens are as big as living rooms, and fitted with islands, Italian tile and massive steel ovens. We spend thousands for top-of-the-line cookware, custom countertops and the latest appliances. We tune in to the Food Channel on cable TV and marvel at the incredible creations of our favorite chefs. Cookbooks that cater to every conceivable taste and style of cuisine can be found among our collection, ready to deliver forth the secret spells of culinary magic.

In an age where even the refrigerator is sentient enough to remind us to buy more milk, what do we do with all of this technology and potential? We order pizza. And on those rare occasions when we really want to "do something special," for our loved ones, we open a can, box or bag with a list of ingredients we can neither pronounce nor comprehend, and nuke the damnable contents in the microwave. This is the state of "cooking" in the 21st century. What happened?

THE GARDEN OF EARTHLY DELIGHTS

Spring in Phoenix, Arizona came quietly to Jefferson Street as it did every year of my youth. The change of seasons in the mild climate of the desert valley, though subtle, was inescapable. The bristly Saguaro in front of Reddy's Corner store would don its spring bonnet of snow-white blossoms while tentacles of Bermuda grass would spread out to reclaim barren patches of dirt from the grasp of winter. Our front yard was a butterfly's heaven in spring, with its Easter palette of fist-sized zinnia blossoms, fragrant roses, and the soft white petals of the oleander bush.

While we got much of our food from the grocery store, we also supplemented our diet with wild catfish and trout, farm-raised chickens, wild rabbit and even deer meat. But of all the ways the working class neighbors of Jefferson Street stretched their meager paychecks, gardening was the favorite.

Gardening in the desert was both a blessing and a curse. The temperate weather meant that you could grow food nearly all year round, but the desert clay was hard and unforgiving. The neighborhood I grew up in was populated by poor people. Few, if any, had anything beyond a high school education. They were all pioneers of the great Diaspora, Africa's children wandering in the wilderness of America. Only two generations removed from slavery, they discovered that life in the North was no easier than it had been in the South, so they migrated West, in search of their own Promised Land. They were Americans in the purest sense of the word, possessed of a strong work ethic and enough optimism to still believe in the messages of pride and self determination delivered in the hand-me-down sermons of Douglas and Booker T. That sense of pride and practicality found expression in the backyard vegetable

45

gardens of nearly every home on the block. While these gardens served the practical purpose of supplementing meager incomes, they were also a source of intense pride that reflected a deep desire for self-reliance.

My mother, a master gardener in her own right, was the goddess Demeter of the neighborhood, coaxing green life from the barren clay of the Sonoran desert. She was a tall woman, heavy set with a stern face and broad shoulders. Her hair was almost straight, jet black and streaked with grey. She loved working outdoors, although I thought she loved watching me and my brother David working more. Mother was from Alabama, a place where the whole world was green. It was there that she learned to garden from her mother. She grew tall stalks of sweet yellow corn, impatient for melted butter and the company of a tender rack of ribs. Deep green collards, honeyed melons and sweet ripe tomatoes too delicious to wash before eating, provided a rich return on the difficult investment of gardening in the desert clay. Grapefruits, tangerines and oranges practically grew wild. Our garden always produced more than we could eat and so we shared our bounty with friends, family and even strangers.

It was in the garden that I learned of the value and rewards of hard work. I saw firsthand the connection between the land and myself, which made the spraying of pesticides on the very food we would be eating unthinkable. In the garden, I practiced the art of patience, as I waited for the warm days of summer and the sweet melons that came with the season. The garden taught me the importance of responsibility when it was my job to keep our dogs out, and the price of irresponsibility when I didn't. When our crop of grapes failed to thrive, even after all our hard work digging, planting and nurturing, I learned that failure and loss are part of living and that we can only do our best, learn from our mistakes and move on.

I would like to be able to say that I have carried these lessons with me all my life, but like many of us, some lessons have been forgotten— or discarded altogether. But a lesson once learned can be relearned and reapplied to one's life. Good food, self reliance, and a love for community, these were the treasures nurtured to fruition by the residents of Jefferson Street. This, their promised land, was a garden of earthly delights.

THE WINDS OF CHANGE

Although my mother was skilled in the growing arts, as time progressed, the food she put on the table reflected the transition we all experienced, from home-grown, home-cooked foods to prepared commercial food.

In the late sixties, we found ourselves in economic peril. My father disappeared from our lives one day and never came back. He had taken these breaks from the rigors of domestic responsibility before and always returned, but this time we would not see him again until his death. Saddled with the responsibility of five children, my mother went to work. She had training as a nurse's assistant, but she could not find such work in Arizona in those less enlightened days, and so became a domestic servant instead.

Our meager income was supplemented by food from a government program which came to be known as the "Commodity Program." Every few weeks, we received a ration of food that included canned spam for meat, powdered milk in a big white box, bottles of clear corn syrup, peanut butter, canned vegetables and dry goods like white flour, rice and pinto beans. On rare occasions, we got cheese.

The corner convenience store a block away from my home was a trove of candy bars and soda pop. We were too poor to afford either on a regular basis, but when we did indulge in these empty foods, it was as a "special treat."

At school, the breakfast and lunchtime menus included cold cereals, waffles, milk, burgers and fries, lasagna and drippy sloppy Joe sandwiches. There's no doubt that the commodity and school lunch programs saw my family through some tough times, but the inescapable fact was that these foods were heavily weighted toward refined carbohydrates, the very foods now blamed for fueling the obesity epidemic.

On the home front, my family's diet slowly transitioned from mostly whole foods to the newer convenience foods. Cheap, store-bought bread that turned to paste in your mouth replaced home-baked bread. TV dinners were cheap and easy to prepare. Adulterated foods that were either deficient in fat or comprised of poor quality fats slowly replaced our dietary staples. Powdered milk, margarine and vegetable shortening were less expensive, more convenient and supposedly healthier than whole milk, butter and lard. We switched to so-called healthy polyunsaturated vegetable oils which we would discover, years later, were highly susceptible to rancidity, making them harmful to the body. Hot oatmeal with butter and whole milk gave way to cold cereals that were nutritionally suspect and packed a wallop of extra carbohydrates and calories. Sugared drinks slowly began to replace milk.

Though not fat, I was a big kid in grade school and feared I would grow fat in time, so I became obsessed with fitness in high school and managed my weight through relentless exercise. Later, the demands of college left me less time to work out and I begin to gain weight. Not much at first, as I still managed to find time to engage in marathon sessions of exercise, but I noticed that despite my efforts, I was beginning to lose ground in my battle to stay trim. By the time I graduated from college and entered the world of work on a full time basis, my processed food diet and the nine-to-five grind conspired to escalate my weight gain dramatically. I didn't realize it at the time, but my struggle with weight gain had begun earlier in my life than that of my parents. My grandparents never had a problem with excess weight.

By the time my own generation came of age, the days of live chickens and barnyard smokehouses had faded from memory. My home and the land upon which it sat were even smaller than my parent's, but cost several times more. Meat came wrapped in plastic from the grocery store freezer, beneath the yellow glow of artificial lights. Half of my meals were eaten outside the home and many of those that were consumed at home came pre-cooked and were thawed and reheated in a microwave. The food I ate came with a cargo of additives, extenders, flavorings and enhancers that didn't even exist in my grandparents' time.

I didn't know and didn't care where my food came from, how it was produced and whether or not the additives were good for me. All I did care about was taste, and the fact that it was it cheap. By the time I reached adulthoood, the only remaining dietary connection between me and my grandparents was gardening.

By the 90s, America had completely bought into the shaky logic of the diet-heart hypothesis which labeled dietary fat and cholesterol as the primary causes of heart disease. We were low-fat and loving it. What we didn't realize was that we had replaced the healthy traditional fats in our diet with vegetable oils and trans fats while gradually increasing our intake of refined carbohydrate foods—the sugars and starches. Parallel advances in technology made our lives physically easier as our cities emptied themselves in a mass migration to the suburbs. We were becoming a nation of sedentary people, spending more time in our cars on the commute to the "burbs" while eating more high-calorie, nutrient-poor foods that rarely satisfied and only left us wanting more.

By the time I became a parent in 1990, I was completely sold on the low-fat, high-carb, convenience food craze. I ate tofu, joined a gym, dieted religiously, became a vegetarian, and still packed on the weight on my way to over 400 pounds. My first daughter followed in my footsteps at an earlier age, gaining weight at an alarming pace after the age of eight.

In our house we had a kitchen, but what usually went on there could hardly be described as cooking. Most of our meals came out of a box, bag or can, or they came by way of a pimply faced kid delivering pizza. Though Mary was gaining weight at a slower pace than I was, she had filled out considerably and no longer resembled the woman I married.

We knew that the problem was with our diet, so we vowed again and again to eat less, cut the fat and exercise more. . . .but it didn't work.

A Life Unburdened

When my second daughter began to get fat at seven years old, Mary and I cursed ourselves for not setting a better example, but how could we? We couldn't help ourselves.

Beginning in the late 1900s through the latter half of the 20th century, two generations of my family lived and died. My generation was still trying to sort fact from fiction amid much conflicting health advice, while my children looked to my wife and me for answers to a problem we had yet to solve ourselves. I looked over the history of my family and I began to see a pattern. As each generation surrendered more and more of its independence to an increasingly industrialized food supply and the corporate kitchen, the less healthy that generation became. As processed convenience foods with their additives and their extended shelf life became the primary source of sustenance for my family, I saw a corresponding increase in weight gain and obesity. Medical problems, from asthma to diabetes, sleep apnea and obesity, were occurring sooner with each succeeding generation.

Despite the progress made in food production, and despite America's miraculous ability to feed the world, in one small corner of that world my family was losing ground. We were more dependent on strangers to feed us, saw our youth interrupted with illness sooner and we were dying at an earlier age.

My parents had been trim and healthy well into their thirties, only succumbing to weight problems later in life. When I was young, two of my four siblings were overweight, seemingly born with a "genetic" tendency toward excessive weight. In my own family, both of my children and my wife were overweight, and I was obese. What was happening to us? It was as though a family curse had been laid upon us, growing worse with each succeeding generation.

On those long nights in New York, when I sat alone in my room, I thought a lot about my family. Dietary chaos reigned on the home front. I felt helpless to do anything about it. What was to become of us? My children were experiencing problems with their health much earlier than I had. Would their lives become a burden for them as well?

Chapter Three

Chaos On
the Home Front

There's no place like home....for gaining excess weight

It is six o'clock in the morning on an overcast day in May of 2003. The northeast business corridor that snakes along the east coast connecting the cities of Boston, New York and Washington D.C., is already alive with commuter traffic. Interstate 95 and the Amtrak rail lines that span the corridor hum like living arteries, sending thousands of morning travelers to points north and south. In one of the outlying suburbs of D.C., my wife, Mary, awakens. Before she can draw her first conscious breath, the feeling that heralds the approach of unwelcome news casts a shadow over her day before it has even begun. Our conversation before I left for New York a few hours earlier was the last thing on her mind when she slipped into a restless sleep. It was the first thought to greet her when she awoke.

We had been sitting together quietly, waiting in the darkened living room, at 3:00 am, for a cab to take me to the train station. I slumped on a sofa facing a large window that looked out onto a deserted street. On these early mornings, our conversations were usually punctuated with intermittent spells of silence. After nearly 17 years of marriage, two children, and an accumulation of over 250 pounds of unwanted body fat between us, we often found there was little to talk about. Lately, these early morning conversations had grown more solemn in tone and seemed to bring the darkness from the outside into our home and into our lives.

"I don't know how much longer I can do this," I said after a long pause.

"Do what?"

"These trips. The job. I just don't know how much longer. . . ." My voice trailed off and faded into the background noises of the house. For a time, the only sounds we could hear were the hum of the refrigerator and my labored breathing.

"Do you have everything, your tickets, your wallet?" Mary was trying to be helpful. She often took this tack when there was a truth she didn't want to face.

"I pick up my ticket at the station," I replied in a lifeless voice. There was another pause. "You need to start thinking about what you're gonna do. . . . when I'm gone."

"What do you mean? You mean today?" She was leaning forward now, but still wasn't taking the bait.

I laughed softly, but there was no joy in my voice. "I mean when I'm gone, gone."

She looked directly at me then. "Richard, what's wrong? Are you OK?"

I inhaled deeply, then coughed as the cool air hit the mucus lying in ambush somewhere along the path to my tired lungs. Another cold had found a home in my worn-out body. I told her about how difficult things had been in New York, told her about the painful days followed by the sleepless nights, told her, finally, about the sense of hopelessness that was slowly drowning me. "I feel used up, tired. I just don't know how much longer I can do this." I choose my next words carefully. "I. . . . feel like I might not be around much longer."

"What. . . ." But she was interrupted by the headlights of the cab piercing the window as it turned into our driveway.

Three: Chaos On the Home Front

I stood up with a grunt and grabbed my travel case. "I'll call you when I get to New York," I said, then kissed her, and stepped out into the dark.

As the tail lights of the cab blinked, then disappeared down the street, Mary began to cry.

Mary was a preacher's daughter. We met in college when I attended her father's church. She had plans to become a doctor. I had seen her before, at the university, usually at the library or the college of science. More than once, I considered approaching her, but I could not tell whether her purposeful stride and serious demeanor were simply the result of a focus on her destination or the outward signs of someone disinterested in consorting with a jock. I wasn't an athlete in the literal sense, but the hours of long distance running, weight lifting, and playing basketball made me look like one.

Mary was different then, too. Despite her modest taste in clothing, which bordered on drabness, she was altogether transformed in church, in hand sown dresses that revealed the supple curves and the muscular sensuousness of a beautiful young woman.

Seventeen years of marriage, two children and an incalculable number of chocolate chip cookies later, she had gained well over 50 pounds since college. But more than the weight that burdened her body was the burden of a life that had not turned out as expected. She had been molested at the age of 12 and left with an emotional wound that had never been allowed to heal. The crime left her withdrawn into a dark corner of fear and self-doubt that manifested in intermittent bouts of emotional darkness, thoughts of suicide and destructive overeating. Our marriage was a series of fights, a scorched earth dotted with frequent brushfires that we could never seem to extinguish for good. They were fueled by Mary's depression and triggered by my quickened temper. More often than not, we doused the flames with food. Food could make you believe you were happy, at least for a short time. Now, medicated on antidepressants, Mary was coping reasonably well emotionally. For several years, life had been better, but the ground she gained in emotional stability was quickly lost in physical health.

MARY'S STORY

In Steinbeck's, *The Grapes of Wrath*, the Joad family pulls up stakes and departs depression-era Oklahoma in search of greener pastures. Mary's mother came of age in the Midwest. Long after the winds of the Great Plains had swept away the dust and dreams of the "Okies," she pulled up her deeply rooted life and went in search of her own green fields. She had fire under her feet and longed to see that part of the world that lay beyond the confining borders of Eufala, Oklahoma.

Unlike her mother, Mary was born and raised in Arizona, and she expected to live there until the end of her days. When I came home one day and told her that my job was moving to the East Coast, she didn't hesitate, having decided that, like her mother, it was time to see a little bit more of the world. With children in tow, we set out for a new life.

That new life was interrupted with a six-month separation while I worked in New York. Mary had been steadily gaining weight for years. In Arizona, she worked as a respiratory therapist and later as a polysomnographer. Both jobs kept her busy and sleep deprived. There was precious little time for cooking and preparing nutritious meals. In her new life as a full time home-worker, Mary wore many hats. She was a mother, home-school teacher, wife, bill juggler, lawn mower, chauffeur, pizza order specialist, food microwaver, and a woman who cried in the dark after the children had been put to bed. Cut loose from the support system she had known all her life, she found herself adrift in a world of indifference and wondered daily how she would cope.

With all the changes and added pressure of her new East Coast life, she soon found herself tilting the scale at 193 pounds. Her doctor tried to be conciliatory, but Mary could sense the doctor's deep concern for her health. She was further troubled by the fact that words like "hypertension," "medication," and "obesity" had begun creeping into their conversations of late, words that she thought would never apply to her.

As Mary's weight gain continued, her health steadily declined. She used to love hiking the rugged desert mountains of central Arizona, but found herself spending more and more time hiking to the refrigerator and the grocery store. She was well on her way to becoming a not-so-proud member of the 200-plus club. She was wearing a size 18 1/2 dress and knew it was only a matter of time before the phrase, "Do you have that in a size 20?" would apply to her.

Moving cross country from Arizona; and the comfortable world of friends and family she had known since childhood, to the cold, alien world that was the East Coast, added a layer of stress to her life that only worsened her physical problems. Now, despite the medication for her depression, the old feelings of hopelessness and despair had begun to return.

THE NEXT GENERATION

The sense of dread had not diminished, when Raven, our youngest daughter, came sleepy-eyed into the room. She climbed into bed and nudged her mother aside. With an impish gleam in her eye, she slipped beneath the covers and settled into the warm spot where Mary had been. This was part of the morning ritual, but it had taken on a new meaning in my absence. Now, a subtle sense of fear seemed to permeate everything. Raven's forays into our bed were a reflection of that fear and the uncertainty she felt at the disruption in our lives with my forced separation to New York. Equally troubling for us were the visual signs of our poor diet reflected in her. Despite the manic energy that seemed to radiate from her, at the tender age of eight years she was gaining weight fast, already starting to thicken around the middle with a miniature alcohol-free version of a middle-aged beer gut. Worse, she was starting to show signs of the same volatile mood swings that afflicted Mary.

Stephanie, our oldest daughter, fared little better. At thirteen years, she was nearly six feet tall. She too was overweight, slow and ponderous for her age. Her complaints of bodily aches and pains were typical of someone much older.

When Stephanie was seven years old, she was diagnosed with precocious puberty, a condition that signals the early onset of physical and hormonal development. The treatment recommended by our doctor involved a monthly hormone injection at the doctor's office. During our visits to the office, I saw the fear in her eyes and held her trembling hand as the long needle bit deep into muscle, sending synthetic hormones coursing through her body. These painful injections, designed to slow her body's blind race to adulthood, left us in a haze of anxiety, fear and doubt. We had questions, but when my wife and I asked about the connection between early puberty and our diet, we felt the sting of the doctor's dismissive response. Eventually, we stopped the treatments against our doctor's recommendation. No one seems to know what causes early puberty, but it has become so common now, that some in the medical community consider the onset of puberty at seven years old to be "normal."

Six years later, we wonder still whether we made the right decision about subjecting her to the treatment. In hindsight, given what we now know about the drug that she was injected with, and food, particularly soy foods and their estrogenic properties that may trigger early puberty, we suspect we made the wrong decision.

In May of 2003, we were a family sinking in a quicksand of health problems. The list of ailments that afflicted us read like a who's who of contemporary disorders: asthma, depression, high blood pressure, poor blood circulation, joint pain, teeth problems, headaches, poor concentration, low energy, insomnia, sleep apnea, acid reflux, and other digestive problems. Through it all, we dutifully took our medications while we suffered, and accepted our various afflictions with heroic stoicism. At the center of these problems was excess weight. As our midsections expanded, so too did the number and complexity of the related illnesses, but this burden of declining health was normal, wasn't it? These things happened to everyone, didn't they?

It wasn't as though we weren't trying to find a solution. In fact, we collected diets the way Tiger Woods collects golf championships. But our scores were considerably higher. In dieting—as in golf—that's a bad thing.

Chapter Four

Dieting in the Dark
An endless search for the perfect diet
leads to places better left alone

When I was in grade school, I developed a keen interest in Greek mythology. One of the most sympathetic characters was Sisyphus. Poor Sisyphus, once employed as King of Corinth, fell on hard times. The CEO of Greek mythology, Zeus, was caught engaging in corporate misbehavior. Sisyphus, overcome by a sense of civic duty, informed on his boss. Unfortunately for Sisyphus, ancient Greece had no whistleblower protection laws, so he was sent to Tartarus, the sub-basement of hell. There he was sentenced to roll a large boulder up a steep hill, but just before he could crest the hill, his strength would fail him and both he and the stone would tumble back down to the bottom. Sisyphus would pick himself up and begin the effort all over again. As there was no parole option available in Tartarus, Sisyphus was condemned to this back-breaking labor for all eternity.

Whenever I started a new diet, I always thought of Sisyphus. The predictable cycle of dieting—success followed by failure—made it easy to identify with his tragic story. When I compared the difficulties of weight loss to boulder rolling, I sometimes wondered whether Sisyphus had the easier of the two tasks.

It wasn't as though Mary and I had not tried to lose weight. Between the two of us, we set off on dozens of dietary expeditions, most of them some variation of the low-fat regimen that most experts recommend.

Looking back, our experiences were a mixture of pleasure and pain, of diets that began with the joy of first-week weight loss but ended in the sorrow of last-week weight gain. Between the hopes and disappointments, we experienced some small victories, but those victories, in every case, were short lived. Long term failure was the overriding theme and the inevitable outcome of all our efforts.

Much has been written about those of us who are overweight and obese. More often than not, we are cast as the villains in life's play. We are the gluttons and idle sinners for whom the selfish quest for pleasure trumps all other concerns. Because we have chosen indulgence, we are judged worthy of scorn and justly sentenced to a life burdened by illness. Of course, most overweight people are neither gluttons nor selfish nor sinners. We do, however, share one virtuous trait; the unshakeable faith that the next diet, the next food fad or the next medical miracle will answer our prayers.

The reason losing weight is so difficult is that most people have very little idea of how to do it. We follow the guidelines set forth by our doctors, the diet gurus, and Aunt Esther, who lost ten pounds in two weeks on the tuna fish and avocado diet, but somehow we never get the results we expect. Clearly there is a disconnect between what is believed about weight loss and what really is true. Until we discover what these truths are, we will forever be dieting in the dark. And so it was with this blind, dogged faith that Mary and I began our own tour of duty in the war against weight.

WEIGHT WATCHERS

I joined Weight Watchers at one point and faithfully attended the weekly meetings. At home, I weighed my food and choked down meals that never quite satisfied my hunger, leaving me in a perpetual state of longing. Still, I had high hopes for this diet. Members met weekly to exchange ideas and encourage each other. The cell I belonged to met regularly in an unassuming strip mall. As an added benefit, I rode my bike the two miles or so to the small storefront office which served as our gathering place. The membership was overwhelmingly female, with only myself and one other gentleman in regular attendance. I don't recall much of what happened in the meetings, beyond the fact that they felt very much like what I imagined a support group should be, only more upbeat. We had public weigh-ins which were only slightly less traumatizing than public executions. There were lively discussions on food, tear soaked announcements of weight loss or weight gain, and spirited transactions in low-fat recipes rivaling anything you might see on the trading floor of the New York Stock Exchange.

While all this was going on, the other man and I sat glumly in the back of the room and inspected our wristwatches. We attempted to talk sports and engage in other y-chromosome conversation. In the end, I grew tired of the recipe exchanges and encouragement intended to make the low-fat diets we were all sentenced to taste better. If these communal gatherings were necessary for success, I saw failure in my future, as I could not see myself at fifty years old, sitting forlornly in a folding chair between two women swapping sugarless, chocolate-free low-fat brownie recipes. I finally made the decision to "go over the wall" when my "cellmate" failed to show up one night. Perhaps if there had been a Men's Weight Watchers I might have lasted longer, but given the typical male's distaste for discussions that touch on personal shortcomings, like a beer gut the size of a VW, I cannot imagine what it is we would have done to fill the time. I don't recall whether I lost any weight while on Weight Watchers, but I did get plenty of exercise riding my bike.

SHAKE, SHAKE, SHAKE

I saw the Slimfast commercials on TV and the ads in the magazines. Here was a weight-loss strategy that did not require attending meetings or participating in public weigh-ins. Slimfast was a powdered meal replacement drink that came in three enticing flavors—vanilla, strawberry, and chocolate. I developed an affinity for strawberry and usually had one for breakfast. At first, Mary joined me in my new ritual of slurping down breakfast shakes, but in no time, she abandoned the faith and left me on my own.

At first, I did lose a few pounds, and although the taste was a far cry from a real strawberry shake, it was not altogether unpleasant. But I soon found that the satiating effect of the shakes was short lived. It was not uncommon to drink one and still be hungry. After a time, it became more and more difficult for me to get by on just a shake as a replacement for a meal. Finally, I just stopped drinking them one day. The partially consumed containers remained in my cupboard for months afterward, a constant reminder of my most recent failure.

THE INFAMOUS CABBAGE DIET

After some initial experimentation, even I knew better than to pursue this one, but the diet had come recommended to Mary by one of her sisters, and so she decided to give it a try. I remember thinking that the diet was remarkably similar to that of starving Europeans during World War II. Mary did not share my passion for history, so she persevered.

To be effective, the diet relied on the prodigious consumption of cabbage as the active weight-loss agent. Adherents were allowed one pitifully small hamburger patty for dinner, but all other meals must consist of cabbage, usually in the form of soup. Mary managed to stick with it for almost two weeks, but eventually succumbed to her body's call for something more substantial. She was quickly reunited with the few pounds she shed. Those pounds brought along some friends from wherever excess pounds go when you lose them temporarily.

THAR SHE BLOWS

The cabbage diet was followed by the tea diet, which was based on an exotic blend of tea containing as its active ingredient a powerful bowel stimulant. The predictable result was akin to launching a nuclear strike against one's colon. This diet had come recommended by yet another of Mary's sisters. Having observed the deleterious effect of the cabbage

. . . .

diet on Mary, I wisely abstained from further participation in unsanctioned human experiments. Mary, ever the explorer, was not dissuaded, and chose to boldly go where no right-thinking person had gone before. Mostly though, she went to the bathroom. The tea left her horribly dehydrated and afraid to eat. The prospect of another Vesuvius-like eruption from her lower regions brought a quick and merciful end to the tea diet.

Mary was one of twelve children and had an inexhaustible supply of sisters. If each one of them had a favorite diet to recommend, I feared for Mary's safety, as there was no telling how much longer she could survive their advice.

THE GYM RAT DIET

While I now knew enough to avoid any diet recommended by Mary's family, I was not deterred from the suggestions of "experts." I decided to follow the guidance of the diet industry gurus who offered the opinion that I was fat because I was lazy and didn't get enough exercise. This flaw in my character was easily remedied, I reasoned, by joining a gym. I signed up with a local gym less than a half mile from my home, and haunted the place both day and night.

Early mornings were not so bad as the place was usually empty and I could exercise on the better machines without interference. Evenings were another story. The happy hour crowd was an eclectic mix of lurkers, stalkers, lycra models and self described ladies men who labored under the mistaken belief that a sweaty fat guy in a jogging suit was somehow irresistibly attractive to well-toned, cellulite-free spandex queens. Taking a cue from Shakespeare, I regarded the whole scene as a grand play—which I took in from my perch atop the stair machine. Often though, I had to wait in line to get a machine and invariably it was my fate to follow the sweatiest man in America, a rolling designation assigned to whoever happened to be on the treadmill or stepper ahead of me.

I was exercising two to three hours a day, putting in punishing hours on the stair climber and the weight machines. The weight fell off so fast that at one point, my gym counselor remarked that I was disappearing before her eyes. This should have been cause for celebration. I was looking like my old self again, but in fact, I was dying inside. The endless hours of exercise were wearing me down. I was bored and tired of living at the gym. I felt as though I had been sentenced to a life of hard labor. If this is what it took to lose weight, I wanted no part of it. Each time I dragged myself onto one of the many medieval instruments of torture, it was a little bit harder than the last time. I was running on the fumes of the willpower I had started with. Eventually, I gave up and promptly regained all the weight I lost, plus—you may have guessed this already—a little bit more.

BETTER WEIGHT LOSS THROUGH SCIENCE

Despite my repeated failures at losing weight, I was not quite ready to give up. I had an abundance of faith in science, and reasoned that if I could not accomplish this task myself, science certainly could. A visit with my doctor was arranged. With the best of intentions, he prescribed a drug, the name of which I no longer remember, but I do recall that the method of operation was reasonably straightforward. Put simply, the drug reduced the ability of my body to metabolize fat. If I consumed more fat than my body could handle—and here the doctor leaned in close as I think he enjoyed imparting this bit of news—the result would be flatulently dramatic and carry unfavorable social consequences. I considered these words for a moment, then concluded that the risk was no less socially acceptable than waddling about at more than one hundred pounds overweight. I was thus undeterred at the prospect of becoming a social pariah and eagerly took the free samples the doctor provided.

I had great expectations for this drug that had as its active ingredient what I came to refer to as "Factor F." To the dismay of a few unlucky and former associates, the drug worked initially. Surprisingly though, in a very short period of time, my body responded to this new chemical assault by somehow overriding the fat-metabolizing limits of the drug and suppressing the flatulence-generating Factor F. In no time, I was popping the pills like jellybeans. Their potency, sufficiently reduced, had little effect on my body. I did not refill the prescription.

THE RABBIT DIET

I would like to be able to say that the rabbit diet was one consisting of variations of cooked rabbit, but that was not the case. Of all the diets we attempted, the most ambitious and initially most promising was our foray into the realm of vegetarianism. I came to vegetarianism with the faith and zeal of a freshly converted sinner. In the beginning, things were great. I felt better than I had in years. I was losing weight and in my own humble opinion, looking great. But the transition was not without its challenges. While I no longer ate meat, I still had a taste for it, a disturbingly strong compulsion that rapidly consumed my every waking thought. And so it was that soy, the miraculous chameleon of foodstuffs, came to my rescue. Having frequented an Indian restaurant that catered to vegetarians, I came to love this pallid lump of flavorless vegetable matter which, with a little imagination—OK, a lot of imagination—somehow made me believe I was still eating meat. I discovered that, like a politician trolling for votes, soy could be anything you wanted it to be.

At the time, the selection of soy-based faux-meat dishes were few, and could only be obtained for a princely sum at a local upscale grocer, the kind that catered to the Jaguar and brie set. At least once a week, I pulled my battered Toyota pickup, with the rattling tail-gate, up alongside the shining Porsches and BMWs in the parking lot, and took my place in the checkout line amidst the affluent class. At least I could rightfully boast to my fellow health-conscious shopping mates that I too was driving an import.

The one thing about soy that troubled me was that it was often used to simulate meat. My decision to become a vegetarian was based on health reasons alone, as I harbored no ethical objection to a slab of prime rib smothered in butter. Nevertheless, I could not help feeling just a little bit hypocritical every time I choked down a soy burger. If eating meat was unhealthy or immoral, why did vegetarians seem OK with pretending to eat meat, and why was I still haunted by this vexing desire for chicken thighs? Was my weakness a sign of a wavering belief in the vegetarian faith, or was I simply experiencing a million years of evolutionary physiological conditioning manifest as the desire to eat what my body needed?

In this brave new world of vegetarianism, where it seemed even the soy products were substituted by others based on soy, I drank loads of skim milk and ate plenty of fruits, vegetables, and sometimes nuts. I also drank gallons of fruit juice, particularly apple juice. Before my conversion, and with the exception of orange juice, I rarely drank fruit juices, as I found them to be too sweet for my taste. But caloric balances, like matter, can neither be created nor destroyed, only changed. So in place of the fat and protein that I once consumed, I substituted prodigious amounts of carbohydrates. This was, after all, the recommended regimen of the dietary experts: increase carbohydrate intake up to 65 percent of daily calories, while reducing fat consumption to 30 percent or less. Most of the fat I did consume came in the form of vegetable oils.

It never occurred to me that despite my weight loss, all those carbohydrates—with very little fat or animal protein—were slowly working against me. I didn't know that many of the carbohydrates I consumed were being converted to fat. I didn't realize that the skim milk I drank was essentially a dead product which provided questionable nutritional benefit. I didn't understand that the vegetable oils and many of the partially hydrogenated fats in the so-called low fat products I consumed were loaded with dangerous trans fats and extra sugar. I had no idea that over-consumption of soy has been linked to breast growth in men, along with nipple discharge and reduced testosterone levels.

Chapter Four: Dieting in the Dark

. . . .

What I did know was that even though I was thinner and looked healthy, I didn't feel healthy. Nearly a year into my low-fat vegetarian ordeal, I found that I lacked the strength to do the kind of physical activities I really enjoyed. I couldn't hike very far without becoming winded. I felt more tired than usual, so exercise was difficult. Once, on a family vacation, I accompanied my mother-in-law on a morning walk that followed a course up a steep hill. She was in her 70s at the time and almost twice my age, but I was the one who had trouble making it to the top.

What was even more troubling was the emotional cloud that darkened my perspective on everything. It seemed to shadow me wherever I went. It manifested itself as a change in mood that lay somewhere between mild discontent and outright depression. The worst of it was my new obsession with food. Every single day, I spent a good portion of my waking hours thinking about food. When would I eat my next meal? How could I doctor up a batch of tofu to make it taste like something edible? If I ate a really big salad, could I fill the hole in my stomach which daily gnawed at me, like an ulcer? What good did it do to fill up on fruits, vegetables and grain products when I was never satisfied and always hungry? I was eating right and living right, so why did it all feel so wrong?

Like my previous failed attempts at losing weight and achieving a healthier lifestyle, this diet too, came to pass. My fall from grace coincided with the death of my father-in-law and an unexpected encounter with a plate of chicken. I was away in California visiting family when the terrible news came. I hurried home to Phoenix to be with my wife who, unknown to me, had gone to comfort her mother who lived some distance away. I arrived at an empty house, exhausted from the trip which had been all the more difficult due to a violent storm that shook up the plane as it descended into Phoenix. By the time I turned the key to the door of our house, I was anxious, saddened by the recent events and extremely hungry. Mary had been entertaining a number of nieces and nephews, all about the same age as my own children, when the news came. There was ample evidence of child's play throughout the house. Not wanting to force our vegetarian beliefs on these children, all of them committed omnivores, Mary had purchased food that was more to their liking, including some fried chicken. I knew from the moment I opened the refrigerator that I was no match for the seductive platter of chicken that greeted me.

I cannot recall how many pieces I ate, only that I abandoned myself to my darkest inner desires. Like the backsliding, meat eating sinner that I was, I wallowed in my crime with a childish glee. All other concerns were forgotten. Each tasty piece of chicken was followed by a solemn vow not to touch another, which was followed by yet one more succulent piece and another vow. Fully satiated, I sat back and patted my much reduced, post-vegetarian stomach, and smiled the smile of the contented. At the funeral, I felt guilty for feeling so good, but the sense of vitality that surged through my body was intoxicating. It took a tremendous amount of self control to keep from grinning throughout the whole affair. Later, the rising tide of newfound energy was so overwhelming, I had to fight to keep from turning cartwheels at the cemetery. It was the first time in over a year I had felt this good. I was alive again, and I liked it.

At first, adding meat to my still mostly vegetarian diet gave me a new lease on life, but having fallen off the vegetarian wagon, I decided to roll beneath the wheels for good measure. Along with the meat, I increased my consumption of unhealthy processed foods full of trans fats, refined flour and sugar. In no time at all, I gained back all fifty pounds I had lost and quite a bit more.

LOW CARB MANIA

I had heard about the low-carbohydrate Atkins diet, but initially wrote it off as just another fad. How, I reasoned, could a man eschew fruits and vegetables, the staples of dieting, and instead gorge himself on meat of every kind and still, somehow, lose weight? As appealing as it all sounded, this regimen made the cabbage diet seem reasonable and prudent. Yet everyday I heard about some new bit of tantalizing evidence that there really was something to low-carb dieting. As the hysteria over the diet continued to build, my curiosity got the best of me. The tipping point in my decision to try it out came as a result of the unexpectedly virulent reaction from the entrenched low-fat camp who all but accused the low-carb converts of trying to commit food-induced suicide. The tenor of the attacks from the low-fat crowd suggested to me that the diet might actually be effective.

Mary and I bought Dr. Atkins' book and read a few chapters—OK we read maybe one chapter and skimmed half of another. We were so excited about trying the diet that we really didn't have time to actually read the book. Eventually, we would pay for our irrational exuberance. We did what I believe many people have done, and simply acted on the information gleaned from stories in the media, the gist of which was that you could eat all the meat you wanted and lose weight, so long as you never consumed any carbohydrates ever again. This advice, by the way, cannot be found in any book recommending a low-carb diet (Atkins recommends lots of vegetables and some fruit, especially after the first few weeks) but back in the heady days of the low-carb craze, this pejorative description of the Atkins diet was all over the local and national news, both in the print and electronic media. So much for accurate science reporting.

The first thing we did was purchase an alarming amount of meat. Beef, fowl, pork, sea food, lamb, it didn't matter really, the only prerequisite being that the day's meal must, at one time, have walked, swam or flown. I imagined that at the height of the low-carb frenzy, barnyards across America were rapidly being depleted of all life. I had a vision of the farm family dog awakening one morning to find all the other creatures gone missing and wondering whether some animal version of the rapture had taken place while he slept.

Our meals took on the look and feel of a Paleolithic buffet where an arugula salad with goat cheese and a light vinaigrette was as rare as table manners at a hunter-gatherer tea party. Had we possessed the knowledge and the means to roast an entire pig and dress him up on a platter with the requisite apple in his mouth, I'm sure we would have done so. I began to feel like a character from *Clan of the Cave Bear*, my contribution to the dinner conversation devolving into rudimentary grunts of, "Meat. More meat."

The amazing thing was that we were actually losing weight. It felt as though we had stepped through a portal into the Bizzaro World of fad dieting, and were living every vegetarian's worst nightmare. Shopping excursions were a breeze. No longer would we tarry for hours in the produce section, squeezing tomatoes and thumping melons. We rejoiced at being set free of decisions about which nutrition-free sugared cereal to buy. Never again would we be disappointed by the pasty, flavorless taste of store-bought refined flour bread. The metallic stench of frozen foods in microwavable bags was now a thing of the past. Our rejection of carbohydrates had nearly freed us from the tyranny of shopping. In the grocery store, we had wings.

But like all bad marriages, our love affair with low-carb dieting went south soon after the honeymoon. Although I never thought it possible, I was actually growing tired of eating meat. On our trips to the grocery store, I would often gaze wistfully, like a rejected lover, at the produce section on my way to the meat locker. My romanticized memories of fruits and vegetables soon turned to lust as my nighttime dreams and daytime visions were filled with shocking images of ripe red tomatoes, succulent fruit, and dark green leafy vegetables beckoning seductively.

To quote T.S. Eliot, the end of our low-carb diet came, "not with a bang, but a whimper." Slowly, our eating habits shifted back to where they once were. Before we realized it, teeth-rotting sodas, fructose-laden, and trans fat-laced foods were once again a part of our lives. It goes without saying that I regained the weight I lost.

I tried dieting, tried exercising for hours each day, tried Weight Watchers, tried diet drugs, vegetarianism and even meatism, but nothing worked. I read books, following the advice of the diet gurus, purchased magazines festooned with bronze hard-bodied cover models and wild claims of "fast, easy" weight loss. After purchasing these magazines and wading through reams of advertising for suspect dietary supplements, I found the claims to be either too difficult to duplicate, suspiciously optimistic or outright dangerous. Along the way, I kept up with the latest weight loss studies and breathless accounts of the most recent "breakthrough," "blockbuster" diet pills touted in the print and electronic media. And yet, all I had to show for my efforts was a closet full of super-sized clothing.

What I and most Americans were unaware of was that beyond the day-to-day concerns of our individual lives during the last few decades, tremendous social, political and economic changes had taken place. These changes would have a profound effect on the health of Americans far into the future. These changes, in fact, are still taking place today. The results can be seen in the staggering statistics that track the growth of obesity, diabetes, cancer and heart disease in this country. It can be seen on the playgrounds of America in the faces of tubby children on diabetes medication, clutching sugary soda pop purchased from the school vending machines.

Much has been said about how to motivate people to make positive change in their lives. I realize now that my failure at weight loss was due not to a lack of sufficient motivation, but to ignorance of the social, political and economic changes that governed American nutrition policy and determined much of what I ate.

Often, I hear from people desperate for change who say, "Just tell me what to do. Tell me what to eat." I do not doubt their sincerity, but I remind them that they are not automatons, mindless machines designed to execute orders without understanding. Real weight loss solutions can only come from a real understanding of the problem and the problem does not begin and end with the individual. Like weeds in a garden, the problem has roots that spread far beyond any individual into the very foundations of our society. Government, industry and the individual all had a hand in creating this problem, and they can have a hand in solving it. A study of the larger reasons behind why we eat and what we eat provided the knowledge I needed to unburden myself of more than 160 pounds.

To begin this study, we'll take a brief look at some of the players who have complicated our efforts to obtain better health. While they are part of the problem, they can also be part of the solution. They are the Diet Priesthood.

Part Two
Losing Our Way

Chapter Five

The Diet Priesthood

Key Players in the Cult of Dieting

Pray for deliverance.

Over the years, I have visited a number of doctors, due primarily to changing health plans and a relocation to the East Coast. Usually during the examination, my doctors avoided the issue of my burgeoning weight, as though my expanding girth was somehow invisible. More likely, they just took it for granted that this was the natural order of things for someone like me, and that they were merely playing their role, writing the requisite prescriptions and offering the cheerless pronouncement that I was "in good health." I always completed that sentence in my mind: ". . . .for someone your size." It occurred to me even then that my doctors were more focused on the symptoms of my problem rather than the root cause: obesity.

Whenever I ventured from the script and inquired about help for weight loss, the invariable response was either to eat less and exercise more or try some new-fangled diet drug that made big promises in the popular press, but offered little beyond scary side effects once I read the fine print. Sometimes I was offered outdated brochures which, given how old they were, may as well have been printed on ancient Egyptian papyrus. Being respectful of professionals in white coats and feeling completely responsible for my poor health, I never bothered to tell any of them that their advice and brochures were completely useless. After all, I knew I needed to eat less and exercise more and I believed that I needed to follow a low-fat diet. But what I really needed to know, the thing that would have been of greatest help to me, was for these learned men and women of science to explain exactly how I was to accomplish these things.

The conclusion I came to over my decade-long struggle with obesity was that all of the reputable experts were pretty much in agreement on the following basic tenets of weight loss:

1. Consume fewer calories than you expend, and you will magically lose weight.
2. Follow a high-carbohydrate, low-fat diet, and you will magically lose weight.
3. Eat whatever you want, in moderation, and you will magically lose weight.
4. Stop choosing to be fat, and you will magically lose weight.

Having followed propositions one and two for years with nothing but additional poundage to show for my efforts, I had little faith in their veracity. Tenet number three was patently ridiculous. How could eating candy bars for breakfast possibly be good for you? If the obese could "eat in moderation," they wouldn't be obese, now would they? As for tenet four, I've never met anyone who wants to be fat. I took this one to be complete and utter nonsense concocted by out-of-touch scientists and policymakers blinded by their own prejudice, a prejudice that equates obesity with sin.

There was something uncomfortably familiar about all this. One day, when I suggested that food might be the cause of a health problem that my daughter was experiencing, her doctor dismissed the notion—and me—with an impatient scowl and a wave of the hand. He would not even entertain the idea. I thought that as a man of science, he might at least consider the possibility, but he seemed positively offended by the notion. It occurred to me that the only other time I had observed this kind of blind faith in one's position was in the area of religion. Religious belief, after all, is based in part on the foundation of unquestioning faith, no matter how illogical the belief.

I began to see in the dietary tenets this same unwavering faith. The truth became quite clear to me. Low-fat dieting was more than just an approach to eating and nutrition, it was an unsound-science-based cult. I realized that there were two types of people who remained true to this faith: the believers, who practiced it, even after years of repeated failure, and those who preached it, the doctors, dieticians, and weight-loss gurus—the diet priesthood.

The diet priesthood is that order of health professionals who seek to preserve the dietary status quo. It matters not that the dietary wisdom of the last several decades has not halted the thickening of America's waistline. Their faith-based beliefs shield them from the unpleasant truth that millions of Americans must live with everyday. When a member of this priesthood is confronted with a notion contrary to what he believes, he will seek to ridicule the idea. When the notion is proven to be true, like the notion that dietary animal fat is beneficial to the human body or that consumption of processed food leads to excess insulin in the body and weight gain, he will denounce the idea while sputtering about the need for "long term" studies and the "increased risks" associated with dietary practices that challenge the status quo.

THE MEDICAL PROFESSION

The medical profession harbors a large number of diet priests. These doctors have abandoned responsibility for patient care to the pharmaceutical industry. Very few received adequate nutrition training in medical school. In fact, some probably understand less about the connection between diet and health than their obese patients. They turn a blind eye to the core cause of obesity—our modern diet—and instead hype expensive drugs and treatments that don't solve the root problem, but only manage and maintain the symptoms, resulting in a steady stream of medical insurance reimbursements and years of suffering for their patients.

Doctors used to look at each patient as an individual with a unique set of problems that must be diagnosed and treated with the appropriate medical solution. No longer. Many doctors today practice a type of treatment model similar to a Paint-by-Numbers hobby kit, where patient treatment conforms to a well established template, whether it works or not. The irony is that some doctors struggle with the very same weight problems as their patients, yet feel compelled to promote a treatment model at which they themselves have failed.

THE PHARMACEUTICAL INDUSTRY

In *The Truth About the Drug Companies: How They Deceive Us and What To Do About It*, author Marcia Angell, M.D., reveals the ugly underside of one of the world's most profitable industries. The pharmaceutical industry leverages taxpayer-funded government research, privatizes it, and then makes billions pedaling their drugs to American consumers at some of the highest prices in the world. Like a virus invading the body of modern medicine, pharmaceutical reps fan out across the country, acting as ghost doctors through their influence on your health care provider. Many doctors naively believe that their prescribing patterns are unaffected by the tsunami of soft money that flows from Big Pharma to Big Medicine. A number of recent studies, along with good common sense, support the allegaton that drug money has influenced the way medicine is practiced in this country, and not always for the better.

These days, sound science and the search for truth compete with the never-ending quest for increased revenues and bigger profits. This trend toward checkbook science contributes to a culture of biased medical research that exaggerates the positive outcomes of medical research, while downplaying or outright ignoring negative side effects.

After college, in the early eighties, I worked as a medical and graphic illustrator for a large hospital in the southwest. One of my duties was to

Chapter Five: The Diet Priesthood
. . . .

assist doctors with developing displays to present the results of their research. These displays typically included poster-sized photographs, illustrations, text and charts. Sometimes the research results for a particular body of work were insignificant. This fact was revealed when blown up to poster size and presented as a chart. It was not uncommon for the doctor to request a reworked chart that exaggerated the increments of the x or y axis in order to exaggerate the research results. This was always explained away as "making the results easier to see." While technically true, we all knew that it was also a way to spin the results to make them appear more meaningful than they actually were.

As factions within the medical industry continue to redefine formerly healthy populations as sick and in need of medication, more and more people are caught up in the net—including children. The ostensible goal is to expand the market for medication to healthy populations previously beyond consideration for drug treatment. Two examples of this trend are blood pressure and cholesterol levels. In both cases, the risk point has been revised downward converting previously healthy people into potential customers for prescription drugs. Crime may not pay, but medicating healthy populations apparently does.

What of the Food and Drug Administration? It is the consensus of many drug industry watchers that the FDA sees the drug industry as a client, rather than as an industry that needs to be watched.

THE FOOD INDUSTRY

The food industry dumps thousands of new products on supermarket shelves each year. To satiate our need for the new and different, (and the industry's need for new sources of profit) the industry inundates us with all manner of laboratory-spawned "Frankenfoods." Once you get beyond the basics of meat, seafood, fruits, vegetables, and dairy, you enter the realm of processed foods. These foods are designed to appeal to our senses with their luxuriant tastes, smells and textures, but beneath their superficial exteriors, they are little more than calorie-dense, nutrient poor "lab experiments" designed to keep us coming back for more.

Under the guise of convenience, the ever expanding prepared-foods sector of the food industry has sold us a bill of goods. With convenience and pricing driving consumer purchases on the buy side, and cold, hard profits driving corporate practices on the sell side, personal health runs a distant third in the race in determining what will be available at the corner store. In short, modern foods have become the real weapons of mass destruction, but unlike their namesakes, they can be found on your supermarket shelf. The American Dietetics Association carries the flag for the processed food industry by promoting the consumption of junk foods as "part of a healthy diet." This is not surprising as the ADA receives funding from several sectors of the processed food industry.

Laws governing the health claims that food industry manufacturers can make have been relaxed under the Bush Administration. As with the drug industry, the FDA rarely intervenes on behalf of the citizens it is supposed to protect. Perhaps it was this industry-friendly environment that contributed to the chutzpah of one popular retailer of fried chicken to air television commercials touting its product as "healthy." Even leaders within the advertising industry—an industry not known for being shy about making outrageous claims—were appalled. The ads were thankfully withdrawn after a short run.

THE RADICAL FUNDAMENTALISTS

A relatively new branch of the priesthood has emerged in recent years, thanks to the Internet. An offshoot, or splinter cell, of the food industry they fulfill the role of attack dog and are more militant in their approach. Like all fundamentalist organizations that employ fear as their primary weapon, these groups engage in wholesale scaremongering to advance their agenda. Funded and supported by legitimate food manufacturers, wholesalers and retailers, these groups operate under jingoistic monikers, with names like "Consumer Coalition for Free Choice," and "Citizen's Group for Freedom." The single tenet of their faith is that infidels, namely anyone who disparages any food as unhealthy, must be publicly ridiculed lest the general public listen to what they say. Their faith requires them to convince consumers that bad people (anyone who disagrees with them) are trying to take away their right to eat whatever they want.

Their writings tend to rely heavily on invectives like "food cop" and "food nanny," and for some reason they are inexplicably fond of the word "tasty," one of those words you don't hear very often outside of the food industry, especially from adults.

THE WEIGHT LOSS INDUSTRY

This group is replete with diet book writers, exercise equipment salesmen and diet supplement manufacturers. Their background in nutrition, diet and human physiology runs the gamut from knowledgeable to laughable. As an example of the latter, not long ago a certain well-known diet guru claimed on national television that the human brain needs 500 grams of carbohydrates per day. Like a puppy working for a treat, a medical expert in attendance eagerly nodded in agreement. Millions of viewers were left ignorant of the fact that the human brain can function quite well with little or no carbohydrates in the diet.

Of all the groups that make up the priesthood, this order is the most flexible. Once they get a sense that money can be made on a new fad, their manufacturing machines are retooled and up and running in no time. Announce on Monday a new study showing that a chemical substance derived from decades-old fruitcake results in weight loss, and the books, CDs, and supplements will be available for sale by Friday.

YOU AND ME

Of course, I can't lay all the blame for our predicament at the feet of government and industry. Sure, we've been fooled, bamboozled, led astray and even lied to by industry and government special interests, but at the end of the day, we are responsible for our own lives. As long as we cling to a blind faith that requires us to accept whatever we are told, we are complicit. When we fail to learn about our own bodies, cook our own food or think for ourselves, we are complicit. When industry says we can eat gobs of sugary, low-fat foods without any ill effect, and we accept that claim without question, we are complicit. When we allow family farmers to be driven off the land and be replaced by factory farms, we are complicit. When corporations and the health care industry bring us the next miracle weight loss drug, and we accept it without question, we are complicit. When we stand idly by as science is co-opted by corporate dollars, and blindly accept the resulting "checkbook" science as sound, we are complicit. And when we allow the food, fashion, entertainment and advertising industries to tell our children what to think, do and be, we are complicit in the demise of our children and ourselves.

THE HERETICS

Fortunately, there are heretics within all of the above groups. These are the unbelievers who go their own way, practicing a Socratic philosophy that challenges conventional wisdom and adheres to the Hippocratic dictate: "First do no harm." They are doctors, medical researchers, nutritionists, authors, food producers and consumers—perhaps even your next door neighbor. Seek them out and support them in their efforts.

A short list of brave heretics includes nutrition researcher, Sally Fallon, author of *Nourishing Traditions*, arguably the best cookbook ever written; Mary Enig, PhD, who tells the truth about fat in her book, *Know Your Fats: The Complete Primer for Understanding the Nutrition of Fats, Oils and Cholesterol*; Uffe Ravnskov, MD PhD, author of *The Cholesterol Myths*; Marion Nestle, author of *Food Politics*, which exposes the Machiavellian politics that gave us our current food policy; and, most important, the late Dr. Weston A. Price, DDS, author of *Nutrition and Physical Degeneration*, for his groundbreaking research on the principles of healthy diets among nonindustrialized people.

Chapter Five: The Diet Priesthood

. . . .

Change is difficult. For some industries and professions, it is downright unprofitable, thus resistance to the idea that conventional dietary wisdom is flawed will undoubtedly continue. Having lost faith in modern dietary wisdom. I have found a new belief system that actually works. That belief system is one based on traditional foods: grass-fed natural meats including organ meats, plenty of animal fats, old-fashioned cod liver oil, wild-caught seafood, organic fruits, vegetables and nuts, whole grains and healthful raw dairy. These are the foods that brought me back from the brink of self-destruction.

Why do we do it? Why do we take on the burden of foods that are clearly unhealthy? Why did we stop cooking our own food? When it comes to our consumer behavior, why do we do the things we do?

Chapter Six

Consumer Engineering and Why We Buy

How we have been trained to buy products and services, whether we need them or not

When it comes to making sense of your shopping behavior, telephones and food have more in common than you may realize. I'll explain in a moment, but first, I want to review one of my favorite children's stories, Pinocchio. Yes, your phone company, the food industry and Pinocchio are all relevant to the question of why you can no longer fit into last year's pants.

In the modernized version of Pinocchio, we have the story of a wooden puppet who wants to be a real boy. The question is, why does Pinocchio want to be real anyway? As a puppet, he can walk and talk and go to school and even learn to read. In fact, in practically every way he can already do what any real boy can do, so what is it that drives Pinocchio? I believe it is the same thing that drives all of us. It has been said that the story of Pinocchio is really about the transition from adolescence to adulthood.

In most versions, Pinocchio is continually manipulated by the characters he meets and these encounters always end in disaster. Very often, Pinocchio is the chief architect of his own misfortunes, but regardless of how he gets into trouble, the one common theme is that Pinocchio lacks the maturity and the ability to direct and control the outcome of his future. That shouldn't surprise us, because he is, after all, a puppet, and puppets have no self control. And while there are no physical strings that direct his behavior, metaphorically, Pinocchio is still bound by his inability to think for himself. It isn't until Pinocchio learns to think and make decisions based on something beyond his own selfish and misguided desires that he is released from his prison of strings. We come to see in a very concrete way that Pinocchio represents all of us and our very human struggle for self determination.

The level of self determination we have—that is, the perceived and genuine ability to chart our own course—is one of the ways in which we judge the quality of our freedom. Few components of social life are more abhorrent than the sense that we are not in control of our own destiny. When we lose this sense of control over our future, we often rebel, but just as often we become paralyzed by hopelessness. Yet the need to be in control of our own lives is so strong that even the illusion of control is preferable to the stark realization that we, like Pinocchio, are mere puppets of a larger, unseen hand that determines our fate.

CONSUMERS MADE TO ORDER

Whenever I talk about the role of consumer engineering in the evolution of how and what we eat, two of the most common responses are shock and disbelief. Some people are shocked at the idea that much of what we know, or think we know, about food and nutrition may not be based solely on the issue of health.

The more common response is disbelief. Some very intelligent people simply cannot comprehend a world in which their thoughts and beliefs about food are not their own. They bristle at the mere suggestion that they may have been manipulated in some way, that their beliefs about food have been engineered as part of some grand, decades-long campaign to make them "better consumers of convenience foods."

In the past, I found it difficult to make a convincing case for the idea that some of our beliefs and behaviors concerning food are, in fact, not of our own making. A task akin to convincing someone who has never seen an elephant that such creatures really do exist. Without an actual elephant, or at least a picture of one, to submit as proof of their existence, incredulity prevails.

Proving the existence of elephants and other oddities of the physical world is quite simple today thanks to the modern miracle of digital photography. But how do you demonstrate to someone that some of their most cherished beliefs such as, "I don't have time to cook," are more a fabrication of clever marketing than a reflection of reality? My mother had five children and my wife's mother had twelve. Both of these women worked outside the home and were extremely busy by even today's standards. How was it possible, then, in an age before the proliferation of microwave ovens, pizza delivery and the avalanche of convenience foods that we have today, that they were able to cook real food and put dinner on the table for their families? Even in the face of these facts, many people still cling to the belief that for the first time in human history, we are too busy to prepare our own food.

The problem, of course, is that we are all victims of consumer engineering. Some of our beliefs about food and nutrition were actually born out of food industry strategy campaigns, in some cases from policy enacted decades ago. Because these changes in opinion took place over a number of decades, it is difficult for many people to perceive them.

I had been searching for a way to describe the phenomenon of consumer engineering when a ride in a cab revealed the solution. The cab driver was a talkative fellow who spent the nearly one-hour ride discussing the foibles of his family. As an example, he told me his wife had given him a mobile phone for his birthday. She had taken advantage of one of those two-for-one phone giveaways that you can't seem to escape from nowadays. The problem was, he already had a mobile phone. What his wife had given him was a new monthly bill, not a gift.

I understood immediately what his wife did not. Though she had saved a few dollars—on a phone her husband didn't even need—her family would be saddled with monthly bill payments. These payments represented an added and unnecessary expense to their household budget. She might just as well have made a voluntary monthly donation to the phone company. From the description that her husband gave, she sounded like a delightful woman, bright and resourceful. How then could she have made such a bad business deal? How did she rationalize her husband's need for a phone when he already had one? Where did she think the extra money to pay for a new phone was going to come from?

On the train, on the bus, on the street, at weddings and funerals, in church and even in public restrooms, mobile phones are everywhere. From eight-year-olds to octogenarians, everyone has a phone these days. If cell phones had existed in the late 1800s, French sculptor Auguste Rodin might well have named "The Thinker" "The Talker," perhaps posing him with a phone cupped to his ear and his mouth wide open.

I've had people tell me they can't live without their phones and more and more people are replacing their traditional land lines with mobiles. Parents all across the country are opening their monthly statements and wailing over their children's three-figure phone charges, then weeping at the loss of their retirement and children's college contributions as they dutifully pay the bill. And it isn't just a matter of technological change: the telecommunications industry is quite literally changing the behavior inherent in communication. Oddly, while mobile phones were supposed to bring us closer together, they are quite literally pulling us apart. I've seen couples on dates where one or both of them are talking on a phone and completely ignoring each other!

How is it that humankind has existed on this planet for millions of years without the need to be in constant communication with each other, while today many people seem practically addicted to their mobile phones? The answer is economics-driven consumer engineering. If you look back just ten short years, almost no one had a mobile phone. How did the telecom industry engineer such a dramatic change in the way we communicate in such a short period of time? They did it through intense and clever marketing. Once you accept the fact that the telecom industry has changed the way we talk to each other in little more than a decade, it starts to seem quite reasonable to acknowledge the fact that the food industry could do the same thing over the course of several decades.

So what are some of the parallels between the two industries? One has to do with cost. Mobile phones are marketed as better, more economic buys, and while it is true that the price of mobile phones has declined steadily, these declining costs only create an illusion of savings. In fact, mobile phones tend to be more expensive due to the complicated pricing structure of the plans, aggressive marketing schemes that package multiple phones and target teenagers, over-consumption of phone services and the often mysterious charges that are included in the typical phone bill.

Much of the same can be said for ready-to-eat convenience foods. While they are generally less expensive than higher quality whole foods, this too is an illusion when you consider the fact that we end up eating more of them. And because these foods are nutritionally poor, any gains in near term economic savings are offset by long-term losses in health, a lower quality of life and the inevitable medical costs.

Here's another similarity: cell phone companies offer an unlimited array of phone models, features and calling plans. Despite this apparent range of choices, the quality of the phones and their performance often fails to meet expectations. Dropped calls, grainy connections and unexplained failures are just some of the unadvertised features of today's mobile phones. Oddly, while they may be quite good at taking pictures and playing MP3s, many of today's mobiles fail to match the connection quality of a rotary dial land line phone from decades earlier.

Convenience foods are similar. While there is much to choose from, the quality leaves plenty to be desired when compared to fresh, whole foods. Much of the decline in quality in convenience food has to do with declining manufacturing standards and an industry obsession with profits. In an era of shrinking margins, how does the food industry convince us to pay for more lower quality food? In a word, marketing.

Ad campaigns for phones often include terms like "free," "most reliable," "flexible," and "unlimited." These powerful words are paired with images of smiling, ethnically diverse groups of attractive people, all enjoying life, ostensibly because of their phones. Now compare those ads with ads for food. Again we find images of happy people bonding at a fast food restaurant while words like "value," "family," "sale" and "quality" complete the implied message: eating certain foods or patronizing certain restaurants will improve your life. We see images of responsible-looking middle class moms who gaze contentedly while their cherub-faced children happily gorge themselves on candied cereals, imitation cheese and French fries. We want to be happy like the people in the advertisements, so we willingly buy the products.

Food manufacturers know that we often base our decisions to buy certain foods on taste, cost and convenience rather than on nutritional quality, and that's what they give us. One of the principle factors that plays into phone purchases as well as food is "image," which refers to how we see ourselves and how we hope others will see us if we buy a particular product. This is standard practice in the world of advertising and should surprise no one, but what is surprising is the degree to which repeated exposure to these messages tends to modify our behavior and shape our opinions. Our opinions should result from our own thoughtful analysis, not from a carefully crafted industry-driven promotional campaign.

For most of the 18 years we were married, Mary and I chose to spend a large portion of our food budget at restaurants and in the purchase of convenience foods. Despite the fact that we were well educated, had only two children, were blessed with flexible working hours, enjoyed all of the technological conveniences of the modern family and grew up in households that cherished the art of cooking, we somehow managed to buy into the proposition that cooking was a tedious and time-consuming affair, one that was beneath our dignity and simply did not fit into our busy schedules.

Fortunately for us, ignorance is only a temporary condition, easily remedied by a willingness to open one's mind and think. We discovered that the reason we didn't cook was because we saw little value in it. Every day, we were directly or indirectly exposed to the message that food purchases should be based on taste, cost and convenience, that we were simply too busy to make intelligent decisions about what we ate, and that we should leave those decisions to the faceless corporations that made things like yogurt in a tube and TV dinners for the microwave. Once we dared to challenge these deeply held beliefs, we realized that the primary factor governing our food purchases should be nutritional quality. Since our parents had somehow managed to provide year after year of delicious meals on a fraction of the income that we had, we concluded we could do the same.

We took a hard look at our beliefs about food and nutrition and found that those beliefs benefited food manufactures more than they did ourselves. We saw that most of the food available at the grocery store was grain-based, filled with sugar and additives, and highly processed. It made business sense for food companies to tout them as better for us and price them so as to make them irresistible.

Why does the food industry resist even a modest effort to provide healthier food? Because that would raise consumer awareness and if even ten percent of consumers switched from buying prepared foods to whole foods, the effect on the food industry would be devastating. In fact, in order to remain viable, the prepared foods industry has to demonize cooking and tell us over and over again that we are simply too busy to cook.

Mary and I soon discovered that we had plenty of time to shop for better quality food and plenty of time to prepare it. It was all a matter of readjusting our priorities. We had surrendered to others the most critical decisions affecting our health. By paying closer attention to what we eat, and by making time for food in our lives, we have freed ourselves from the burden of poor health. Just like Pinocchio, we have refused to be misguided by others, and instead have learned to recognize the value of real self-determination.

Chapter Seven

The Trojan Horse Diet
What if some of the "healthy" foods you're eating
are doing you the most harm?

We owe a great debt of gratitude to Dr. Weston A. Price for his contribution to the study of human nutrition. Dr. Price was a dentist who in the 1930s and 1940s traveled to remote areas of the globe and discovered key principles of traditional diets. As a dentist, Dr. Price was principally concerned with the connection between diet and dental health. What he uncovered was the connection between the increasing industrialization of the food supply and the physical degeneration of the populations who consumed this food, manifested as rampant tooth decay, narrowed jaws and crooked teeth (what he called "dental deformation") in the next generation.

Accompanied by his wife and the occasional guide, his travels took him from isolated Swiss villages nestled in the Alps, to hardy communities of Eskimos in the wilderness of Alaska. In Polynesia, Africa, Australia and many other out-of-the way communities, he discovered the same connection between food and health. In a general sense, his discovery can be summed up quite simply. When isolated people adhere to their traditional diets, their health and quality of life is much superior to their condition after adopting a modern diet high in refined grains, sugar and other processed foods. The problem gets worse with succeeding generations that grow up on a modern diet. They experience advanced tooth decay, physical deformities, a loss of overall vigor, decreased resistance to disease and a lower quality of life. Dr. Price documented his research in his book, *Nutrition and Physical Degeneration*, a stunning account—in words and pictures—of what happens when diet goes awry.

A key finding of his research was that foods like liver, organ meats, fish eggs, fish liver oil and eggs and butter from pastured animals contained high levels of vitamins A and D. These life-giving foods are the very foods now condemned by the diet priesthood.

The physical degeneration that Dr. Price observed in the first half of the last century began with the advent of processed food and continues even today. In fact, the rise in chronic diseases associated with civilization—heart disease, diabetes, obesity and cancer—plague us in even greater numbers today, despite our advanced knowledge of human physiology and the slew of drugs and treatments we use to control them. This rise in chronic disease exactly parallels the increasing industrialization of our food supply.

Of course, environmental pollutants and destructive lifestyle choices also play a role in our declining health, but the foods we eat, the foods that literally become a part of us, are the primary contributors in the breakdown of the human body. Our modern diet of processed, easy-open, labor-saving, pre-cooked, just-add-water, fat-free convenience foods seem like a miracle at first glance. We have been freed from the "tyranny" of cooking, but at what price?

FACTORY FARMS

In 1906, American writer Upton Sinclair published *The Jungle*, a scathing exposé of the American meatpacking industry. Sinclair's vivid portrait of unsanitary and morally bankrupt slaughterhouse practices brought about sweeping changes within the meat industry. We can all breathe easier now knowing that the corrupt practices of early 20th century America are behind us—or can we?

Our meat is cleaner today than it was in Sinclair's era, but what do we really know about where our food comes from? Advertisements for dairy products show contented cows lolling in verdant fields of clover, beneath tranquil blue skies. Promotions for meat products often avoid showing the actual animals, lest we accidentally make the connection between that cute calf or pig, and the pork chop or slice of veal on our dinner plate. For several generations now, we have been literally and figuratively cut off from our food, but as we've learned, it wasn't always that way.

Today's factory farms engage in the kinds of practices Upton Sinclair wrote about. Dairy cows are held in confinement conditions and forced to stand on concrete floors their whole lives. They live in cathedral-sized metal sheds that epitomize man's inhumanity to animals. They are fed an unnatural diet of grain, soy, bakery waste and swill from ethanol production to keep the milk flowing. The cows have been bred to have enormous udders bio-engineered to deliver far more milk than Mother Nature ever intended. Growth hormones like BST (bovine somatotropin) are used to stimulate higher levels of milk production. Not surprisingly, these animals get sick often, and are kept "productive" courtesy of a strenuous course of antibiotics. One particularly nasty illness called mastitis, an infection of the udder, is pandemic in the confinement dairies. The infected animal may secrete pus in its milk resulting in a substandard product that must be filtered and pasteurized before your child can drink it with any assurance of safety.

Pigs and chickens have not been excluded from the mistreatment suffered by cows. Pigs are held in confinement conditions so stressful that they engage in the practice of chewing each other's tails. Industry's response to this problem is not to reduce the number of pigs on a farm, or increase the acreage to accommodate them, but to chop off their tails! Meanwhile, biochemists are trying to breed the stress gene out of the pigs so that they'll suffer their fate in stoic silence.

Industrial agriculture has turned chickens into egg-laying machines, confined in cages with barely enough room for them to move around. I have found the taste of chicken today to be remarkably inferior to that which I recall as a child. In those days, the meat was firm and flavorful and the bones quite hard. Today, meat from grocery store chickens is distastefully mealy, and the bones disturbingly soft. The commercial eggs have pale anemic yolks, inferior in taste to the delicious, deep-yellow-colored yolks of the eggs from pastured chickens on a more natural diet.

Besides the illness and stress these animals suffer, the humans who live with and near them must deal with another problem: what to do with all the waste? As you might imagine, the accumulated waste produced by too many animals in too small a space produces smells so bad it makes people sick. The waste is held in onsite containment ponds. A recent news article describes how the wall of a containment pond gave way, causing a massive spill. Thousands of gallons of putrid sludge poured into a drainage ditch and eventually made its way into a nearby river, killing thousands of fish.

Factory farming taints everything it touches: animals, farm workers, food, and those who consume it.

THE MODERN TRADITIONAL DIET

The healthy indigenous people that Dr. Price studied consumed a traditional diet devoid of refined and processed food. What constitutes a traditional diet? Today, many children begin their lives on soymilk before graduating to soda, sometimes while they're still on the bottle. A traditional diet does not necessarily mean, then, the first food you eat. To delineate a traditional diet we must first define the word "food." Eating wisely requires us to know what is in our food and what effect it will have on our long-term health. We also need to distinguish between "food" and "real food." Generally speaking, most people define food as anything we eat for nourishment, energy or the simple desire to satisfy our taste. This is a broad definition, as you'll see, because people are remarkably adaptable with regard to what they'll eat.

I knew a kid in grade school who was particularly fond of paste. He would snitch great gobs of the stuff and eat it surreptitiously when the teacher wasn't looking. In some parts of the world, eating dirt is not uncommon. Some people have even been known to consume unlikely objects, like nuts and bolts. Most of us would not consider paste or a three-quarter inch lug nut as food, so let's refine our definition a bit more.

Food is any edible substance originating from a natural plant or animal source, which is consumed for the purpose of providing nourishment and energy. This is a better description, but let's examine this further. *Real* food is food that has been minimally processed and retains its natural life-giving properties. Most of the added ingredients in our food are completely unnecessary for proper human nourishment. In some cases, they may even be harmful. These additives exist for three reasons, none of which has anything to do with nourishing the human body. The first is to mimic freshness by artificially extending the shelf life of the food. Without these additives, many foods would go stale and rot. The second reason is that many commercially produced foods simply don't taste very good, so additives are used to enhance flavor as well as visual appeal. The third is that manufacturers are always looking for ways to cut costs and increase profits. Artificial food additives reduce cost by replacing real ingredients with fake ones. Generally speaking, the fewer additives and preservatives a food contains, the more real it is.

The process by which foods are produced also determines how real they are. Beef from a cow that has been raised in abusive conditions on a diet of grains, growth hormones and antibiotics is not the same as beef from a grass fed, healthy cow. Packaged foods that have been sterilized, synthesized, homogenized, colorized, pasteurized, emulsified, flavorized, pulverized, deodorized, irradiated and genetically modified do not qualify as real food. Artificially flavored and colored "yogurt" that does not require refrigeration and comes in a squeezable tube is an extreme example of this type of not-real food. "Beef" ribs made from soy is another.

A Life Unburdened

. . . .

Manufacturers are the primary beneficiaries of this type of food production. Consumers lose because eating foods comprised of substances that are foreign and possibly harmful to the human body, and produced in a manner inconsistent with good nutrition, ruins our health.

Real food, then, can be defined as food that contains few or no additives or artificial ingredients. Real food nourishes, builds and energizes the body, and is produced in a manner consistent with retaining the life-giving properties of the food. Everything from salads to pizza made from real ingredients qualifies as real food. These are the traditional foods that have nourished humanity down through the ages. It follows, then, that a traditional diet is one comprised of real foods that are in harmony with the evolutionary physiology of the human body.

A DIETARY ODYSSEY

Two of my favorite stories growing up were Homer's twin epics, the *Iliad* and the *Odyssey*. They tell the story of the long and difficult Trojan War, and of the Greek hero, Odysseus' even longer journey home. I was especially fascinated by the Trojan horse, a "gift" from the Greeks that turned out to be the instrument of the Trojans' defeat. Today, poor dietary advice has turned out to be a Trojan horse in the lives of many unsuspecting people. For decades, we have been at war with our cultural and culinary history in our rejection of dietary fat and traditional foods. Fat, particularly saturated fat, has been the scapegoat for all that is wrong with what America eats. The oft repeated warning to "eat low-fat," has become more than just a cornerstone of nutritional dogma—it has become sacred scripture, forever in the minds and upon the lips of the diet priesthood and millions of faithful adherents.

We have adopted a nutritional belief system that demonizes fat with the fervor of religious zealotry. It is a faith we practice daily, making fat-free food choices with a numbing sense of duty that approaches fundamentalist fanaticism. We have been taught that salvation and thin thighs can only be attained by a strict adherence to a fat-free lifestyle, and so, without question, we blindly submit our bodies, our minds—and our children—to this belief.

Yet despite an almost universal belief in low-fat dieting, most of us succumb to weight gain, illness and premature death. Although obesity, heart disease, diabetes, allergies, asthma and fatigue befall us, we soldier on, obediently invoking protection against the evil of dietary fat, while we medicate ourselves into oblivion.

WHAT ARE WE REALLY EATING?

The image of Americans as lazy gluttons stuffing themselves with prodigious amounts of dietary animal fat is a gross exaggeration of the truth. The following statistics from the *USDA Food Consumption, Prices, and Expenditures* report reveals what Americans really eat. Except where noted, the report covers the period between 1970 and 1997.

Although per capita consumption of meat of all types reached near record high levels in 1994, the proportion of fat from meat declined from 35 percent in 1970 to 25 percent in 1994. Saturated fat consumption fell from 37 percent to 26 percent. In 1960, beef producers began raising leaner beef by moving away from the traditionally fatter and tastier breeds, like Herefords and Angus. The trends are similar for pork. While overall consumption increased slightly from 1970 to 1998, the meat was much leaner, reflecting the consumer trend toward low-fat eating. In total, per capita meat consumption, including red meat, poultry and fish, was up about 13 pounds per year, but this change was due mostly to an increase in poultry consumption. Consumption of red meat, which was significantly leaner and contained much less saturated fat, declined.

Shell eggs, once considered a perfect food, saw a per capita decline from 276 to 173 eggs from 1970 to 1997, due to consumer fear that the cholesterol in eggs causes heart disease. Between 1970 and 1994, per person consumption of cholesterol declined 13 percent, from 470 to 410 milligrams. Yet heart disease remains at epidemic levels.

In the dairy category, whole milk consumption decreased by two-thirds between 1970 and 1997. This decrease was offset by America's love affair with cheese and fluid cream products. Average consumption of cheese increased 146 percent! Lest you think Americans inexplicably evolved into connoisseurs of fine gourmet cheeses, think again. Most of that cheese—up to two-thirds—came packaged as convenience food in the form of pizza, snack foods, fast food sandwiches, chips, bagel spreads, etc. While cheese is a high-fat item, when it comes as convenience food, it is accompanied by prodigious amounts of grains and sugars. Consumption of fluid cream products (heavy cream, light cream, sour cream and other dips) increased from 9.8 half-pints to 17 half-pints, while overall fluid milkfat consumption (whole and reduced-fat milk and cream) declined by 37 percent.

Surprisingly, in 1997, Americans, on average, consumed 57 pounds more fruit and 87 pounds more vegetables than they did in 1970. Given all the finger wagging from health experts, you would never guess that produce consumption has risen so much.

The most startling figures in the report come in the grain, sugar and fat categories. Americans' consumption of flour and cereal products increased from 136 pounds in 1970 to a whopping 200 pounds in 1997. That's a lot of dough. Much of this increase came in the form of fast food and snack food such as pizza, pasta, crackers, chips and—the mother of all grain foods—ready-to-eat cereals. Breakfast cereal consumption between 1980 and 1997 increased by 41 percent to 17 pounds per person per year! Much of that cereal was consumed with mounds of sugar. In fact, in 1997, our consumption of sugars—table sugar and high-fructose corn syrup (HFCS)—rose 28 percent, or 34 pounds per person, for a total of 154 pounds of the sweet stuff. That's 53 teaspoons per day! A far cry from the 6 to 18 teaspoons (based on a diet of 1,600 to 2,800 calories) our government recommends in the Food Guide Pyramid. The use of corn sweeteners, especially HFCS, skyrocketed due to favorable government agricultural policies toward corn growers and an overabundant supply. One place these corn sweeteners wound up was in beverages. In 1986, the average American swilled 28 gallons of carbonated soda. By 1997, that number had increased to 41 gallons, a

47 percent increase. Soda has replaced milk as the drink or drug of choice among children and teenagers.

Finally, let's look at fats and oils. Unless you live in a whole foods commune, it's unlikely that you know anyone who cooks with lard, tallow, coconut or palm oil. Even the use of butter is a rarity today. Between 1970 and 1997, consumption of animal fats declined by a fourth while consumption of polyunsaturated vegetable fats increased by two-fifths. During this same period, consumption of polyunsaturated salad and cooking oils jumped from 15 to 29 pounds per capita! Experts like Mary Enig, PhD, have warned the public about the fact that polyunsaturated vegetable oils can become oxidized quite easily, forming free radicals that cause cancer and atherosclerosis in humans. Unfortunately, health "experts" have been advising us to consume polyunsaturated oils as a preventative measure against heart disease and cancer since the 1950s. These rancid oils are, in fact, more likely to create health problems than prevent them. Government policy also promotes consumption of partially hydrogenated vegetable fats which are engineered to behave like saturated fat. These fats, in the form of margarine and shortening, are loaded with harmful trans fats. Baked goods, including cookies, cakes and crackers, peanut butter, fried foods, soups and cereals are all loaded with trans fats. Commercial salad dressings contain both liquid oils and partially hydrogenated oils. We eat far more of these dressings today than we did 30 years ago because we are following the advice to eat more salads! A USDA survey showed that between 1989 and 1991, the average woman between the ages of 19 and 50 obtained more vegetable fat from salad dressing than anything else she was eating.

A Life Unburdened

. . . .

Changes in U.S. Per Capita Food Consumption, 1970 - 1997

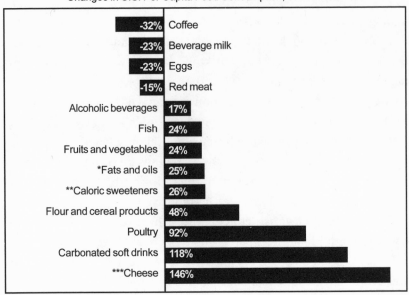

Source: USDA Economic Research Service
*Represents added fats and oils (shortening, margarine, vegetable oil, butter) found in fried foods, snack foods, and salad dressing. Excludes natural fats found in foods like milk and meat. By 1994, these fats and oils contributed to 52% of total fat intake. Meat, fish, and poultry followed with 25% of the total.
**Includes caloric sweeteners used in soft drinks.

***Two-thirds of cheese consumption came in the form of prepared foods

Trends in Obesity from 1976 - 2000

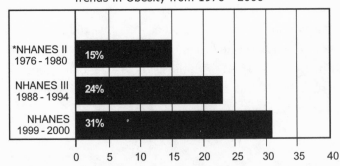

Source: Derived from the CDC and the National Center for Health Statistics
*National Health and Nutrition Examination Survey
Age-adjusted by the direct method to the year 2000 U.S. Bureau of the Census estimates using the age groups 20-29, 40-59, and 60-74 years.

Chapter Seven: The Trojan Horse Diet

. . . .

OBESITY AND HEART DISEASE

It is interesting to note the changes in the health of Americans over the same time period as the food consumption survey. According to the 1999-2000 National Health and Nutrition Examination Survey conducted by a division of the Centers for Disease Control, rates of obesity doubled between 1976 and 2000. Heart disease continues as the number one killer in America, racking up 945,836 lives in the year 2000, according to the American Heart Association. While the death rate from heart disease has declined slightly, due to improvements in treating the disease, Americans continue to be stricken by this killer in astounding numbers.

When I look at these statistics, I see a reflection of myself. Just like many other Americans, I followed the prevailing health advice. I ate more fruits and vegetables and less fat, and abandoned whole milk and eggs. I cut out most red meat and substituted poultry, cooked with polyunsaturated oils and replaced butter with margarine. I consumed prodigious amounts of sweetener in soda, fruit juices and just about 90 percent of the convenience foods on my grocery store shelf. I didn't smoke, drink alcohol or coffee. In short, I did just about everything the experts said I should, but despite my virtuous life, I still managed to gain over 200 pounds.

What I didn't know was that the polyunsaturated vegetable oils and partially hydrogenated fats that had replaced the animal fats in my diet were destroying my health. I didn't know that my low-fat diet was actually fueling the appetite to eat more. I never realized that a diet high in grains, sugars and supposedly healthier vegetable oil was actually a Trojan horse, putting pounds on me faster than I could exercise them off. I didn't know that the reason I failed at dieting so often was because the food I ate was grossly insufficient in meeting my nutritional needs. I didn't know that bingeing and devouring an entire family-sized bag of potato chips was a sign that my body was craving healthy fat. I didn't know that those late-night eating marathons could have been completely ameliorated had I simply added a little healthy fat in the form of a steak, some coconut oil or butter to my diet. In the end, I didn't know that my inability to exercise regularly had more to do with a series of diets insufficient to sustain me physically and mentally. There was a lot I didn't know and apparently, none of my doctors knew anything either.

Dietary animal fat has been pegged as the primary culprit in the long-running siege against our health. However, when you review the USDA statistics, you can see that while consumption of saturated fat has decreased overall, consumption of processed convenience foods has increased dramatically. Is it really that difficult to see the connection between these foods and the increase in heart disease, obesity and diabetes?

It has been well established that obesity is a risk factor for heart disease. As many consumers have embraced low-carbohydrate dieting, our government has sponsored a number of studies intended to refute low-carb dieting. Instead these studies proved the truth of the connection between excess refined carbohydrates and obesity. Is it not reasonable to suggest that heart disease, which correlates with obesity, may be connected to our increase in consumption of non-traditional fats as well as the excess starches and sugars found in processed foods? Why then does the scientific community continue to obsess over saturated fats?

I don't mean to suggest that the Western diet is the sole cause of heart disease. Smoking, stress and physical inactivity play key rolls as well. What I do suggest is that there are many questions that directly challenge the validity of the theory that cholesterol and saturated fat cause heart disease. So many questions, in fact, that one begins to wonder where, exactly, is the science behind the theory? It almost seems as though the proponents of the diet-heart hypothesis are operating more on their personal faith in the theory and less on scientific fact. Despite their protestations in favor of "sound science," they are little more than faith healers themselves.

As the truth about dietary fat emerges, and we begin to reapply the wisdom of our ancestors, we can celebrate a long awaited homecoming. Like Odysseus, the road home to wellness may be long and difficult, but Odysseus made it. I found that once I mustered the courage to plot my on course home, I could make it, too.

THE DIETARY DARK AGES

For the last few decades, I've lived through a personal and public Dark Ages of nutrition and health. I have witnessed—with my own eyes— a steady increase in obesity, an increase in the incidence of adult disorders in children and an increase in unexplained cancers. The answer to the question, "How did this happen?" was not easy for me to accept. I had to let go of much of what I thought I knew about nutrition, exercise and public health policy. I had to open my mind to some old and some new ideas.

The good news is that Mary and I discovered that the story of our lives does not have to follow the script that was written for us. Even better is the news that you don't have to be an expert to change your life and improve your health. We did just that, losing more than a combined 200 pounds without doctors, drugs, dieting or surgery. The best news of all is that losing weight was just the beginning of a physical and mental transformation that changed the way we see the world and ourselves. It's why I wrote this book. But before I tell you about how we changed the direction of our future, I have to tell you how we put the breaks on our past. The amazing thing is that I owe this life-changing experience, this personal reclamation, to an order of take-out chicken.

Part Three
The Road Home

Chapter Eight

An Epiphany and a Plate of Chicken

How could something as simple as a take-out order of chicken save a man's life?

In 2003 I was on a temporary assignment, living and working in New York City from January through May. I lived out of a suitcase in Manhattan throughout the week, returning home to Virginia on the weekends. I found myself under considerable stress and ate every meal, nearly five days a week, at either a sit-down or take-out restaurant or through room service. In between restaurant meals, I snacked on whatever was available.

My weight, already at a level that would have landed me a salaried position with a traveling circus, now rocketed into the fatosphere. I suffered the usual obesity-related ills: back and joint pain, difficulty walking, shortness of breath, headaches and fatigue. My daily intake of food fluctuated between 5000 and 7000 calories. In New York, finding a place to eat is never a problem. Add work-related stress, calorie-dense foods and the heroic proportions served in most restaurants, and maintaining a stratospheric calorie count is really quite easy. In addition, I drank gallons of fructose-laced soda at 25 cents a can and launched nightly raids on the snack bar that haunted my hotel room. I was a walking cautionary tale on the evils of gluttony, an accidental Frankenstein's monster cobbled together from the rubbish heap of processed convenience foods, and dietary ignorance.

A Life Unburdened

. . . .

I realized my diet was a key factor in my declining health, so one day I decided to go on a 24-hour fast. I was only partially successful, as the familiar craving to eat, heightened by a series of Pavlovian triggers, drove me to break my vow and grab some dinner. I found myself at my favorite carry-out deli in lower Manhattan, a little place with the unusual name of the Lord's Deli. I wanted something light, a salad maybe, but the menu mostly featured heavily sauced dishes of pasta buried beneath pounds of melted cheese so there was little to choose from. Even the pan of sautéed vegetables came smothered in a vat of oil. I finally chose a small portion of roasted, skinless chicken breast, accompanied by the vegetables which I planned to rescue from their hot oil bath once I returned to my hotel room. The chicken, infused with herbs and butter, was delicious. That night, I drank water with my meal, instead of soda, and fell into a restless sleep.

The next morning, I felt better than I had in weeks. I had a light breakfast and skipped lunch, saving myself for a repeat of that heavenly chicken. I ordered it again the second night, two pieces this time, and skipped the veggies. The next morning, I was beginning to feel like a changed man. When I walked to work, my back pain was nearly gone. I found that I had more energy and even my normally sour disposition had improved—approaching something that could be described as "sunny." This was all good news, but I couldn't see myself eating nothing but roast chicken for the rest of my life.

It was at that point that I had my epiphany. What if the changes I was experiencing had more to do with what I was NOT eating? For two days I had had no glutamates, no cyclamates, no nitrates, sugar, soy products or refined carbohydrates – in short, no processed food.

A REVELATION ON THE HOME FRONT

Two hundred miles away in Virginia, Mary was having a similar revelation. She had received a phone call from her sister, Kathy, with news of an uncle's death. As they were exchanging goodbyes, Kathy remarked on how good she and her husband had been feeling lately.

Chapter Eight: An Epiphany and a Plate of Chicken

She talked about how they had lost weight and had a surplus of energy. Hungry for some good news, Mary asked her what was it they were doing.

"We're just eating the food we grew up with Mary," came her reply. She continued, "We stopped eating all that processed food." There was a pause. "We eat eggs Mary, and butter, too."

"Butter? Eggs!" Mary was in shock.

"Don't be afraid of eggs," Kathy said, "They're good for you."

Their conversation continued a bit longer, with Kathy providing the titles of some books that she had been reading which had triggered this new attitude about food. Mary was mesmerized. It was too good to be true. She quietly dropped the receiver into its cradle and for a moment sat with her hand resting on the phone. Then, her mind made up, she called both of our daughters.

She addressed them as an officer to the troops. "Girls, things are going to be different from now on. The first thing we're going to do is get rid of all this junk food we have in the house. We're going to start cooking our own food. . . ." she paused, gathering her courage, "and we won't be ordering any more pizza—and there won't be any more soda either. We're going to start eating normal. . . ." she groped for the right words, "regular food, like I used to eat when I was a little girl."

The girls exchanged alarmed glances. This sounded serious. Mary went on to explain her decision, as best she could. She had that dead-serious, determined look on her face that meant that there was no room for negotiation.

And so commenced what came to be known as the "Purge." With trash bags in hand, any food item that failed to pass the test for authenticity was snatched up and consigned to the trash. The test for authenticity was quite simple. If an article of food contained ingredients that required a laboratory and people with advanced degrees in chemistry to replicate, it failed.

I called Mary a couple of days later to tell her how much better I felt and was surprised—delighted—to hear that she had come to a similar conclusion.

A Life Unburdened

On June 1st, 2003, we embarked on what would eventually become a whole foods way of eating. I had dieted before. I knew the chance of failure was very high, so I decided to do something different this time. Let me say that again, because that moment of clarity represented a turning point in my life: "I decided to do something different this time."

Albert Einstein said, "The definition of insanity is doing the same thing over and over again and expecting different results." For over a decade, I had followed the same course of action: adopting a new diet, sticking with it for a time before collapsing into my old habits, then regaining any weight I had lost, plus a few bonus pounds for good measure. In every case, I had faithfully followed the rules, resulting in a little success in some cases and a lot of success in others, but the end result was always the same. Failure. I realized that in every case, I actually had very little understanding of why the diet worked or didn't work, had no idea of how the human body metabolizes food. I was simply doing as I had been told by the dietary experts: "Eat a balanced diet and get plenty of exercise." The problem with this advice was that that it had never worked for me. I mean, if I knew what a balanced diet was and was able to stick to it, I would not have had a weight problem to begin with.

I decided I would not commit the crime of "just following orders," as I had done so often before. This time I was going to find the answers for myself. If a whole foods diet really worked, I wanted to know why. I wanted to see the studies that proved it, wanted to uncover the metabolic processes behind it. So I began to read and as I read, I discovered just how convoluted America's nutrition policy really is. I came to see why my doctor had never been able to give me any useful advice when it came to weight loss.

I plunged into the history of nutrition politics in America and came up reeling. I read *Food Politics* and *Safe Food*, by Marion Nestle, *Fast Food Nation*, by Eric Schlosser, *Fat Land*, by Greg Critser, the *New York Times* article *What if it's All Been a Big Fat Lie*, by Gary Taub, and countless other articles, position papers and medical research reports. I looked to the sciences for relief, and found that in this area too, human pride, prejudice and greed have forever tainted what has become the flawed dietary policy that millions of Americans follow. I began to see, for the first time, the folly of a medical industry that expends innumerable resources on the treatment of obesity-related symptoms, but adopts a hands-off approach when it comes to treating the source of those symptoms: poor nutrition.

I marveled at the zealous adherence to the religion of low-fat eating when there is clear evidence that for most people this approach does not work. I saw manipulation by powerful industry groups that influenced what I and my children ate, learned how corporations subvert parental authority by spending millions on child psychologists and sophisticated advertising campaigns in an aggressive effort to market junk food directly to our children on television, and in the schools. I saw how this influence is exerted on the people we look to for leadership, from doctors corrupted by pharmaceutical industry largesse to ethically conflicted scientists, politicians and bureaucrats—saw how economics played and continues to play a critical role in shaping nutrition policy and in misshaping us.

In time I came to realize that the mantra of personal responsibility, intoned by representatives of the food industry and their friends in government, is true, but not in the way they intended it. Real personal responsibility means looking past the dogma promulgated by industry interests for their own benefit. As a practical matter, it means learning about basic human physiology and the mechanics of food metabolism. It means adopting an unapologetically discriminatory mindset when it comes to deciding what you put into your body. It means skipping the marketing hype on the front of food packages and reading the ingredient labels on the back. It means learning to identify industry-influenced "journalism" masquerading as unbiased health and nutrition reporting that appears in our newspapers and magazines. It means acquiring the language of the scientist to decipher the double-speak and disinformation often employed to hide the real results of industry-sponsored studies on health and nutrition issues.

In my journey, I've discovered that the one-size-fits-all model for diet and nutrition advice does not work for me and does not work for most. I learned that focusing on just one food group is a mistake; that the experts really don't know as much as I thought they did and that they are not telling me everything they do know. I realized that I needed to question all that I knew, or thought I knew, about nutrition.

TIME FOR A CHANGE

In June of 2003, I returned home to my family for good. My work on the New York project was over. I took this as a positive sign that it was finally time to make a real change. In the span of just one week, my change in diet from processed to whole foods had already worked a miracle. Suddenly, I had more energy and optimism. I was no longer just plowing through my day, trying to make it through to late night TV. I had a purpose now, and each new day provided an opportunity to make progress. Where did all this optimism come from?

I realized my diet weighed me down in ways that I had not expected. When you think about it though, it shouldn't come as a surprise that food exerts a mental and emotional effect, as well as a physical one. That effect can be a burden or a blessing. Our bodies are just chemical factories after all. It was a good thing I had so much optimism, because I would come to learn that I would need every bit. Now for the details of how we got started on our journey and how we stayed the course.

Chapter Nine

The Road Home
Coming back from the brink of oblivion

The buzz of the alarm clock roused me out of a shallow sleep and left me blinking into the dark. I had awakened a half hour earlier and spent the last 30 minutes moving gently between the dreaming and waking world. I pulled off the covers and in one motion swung toward the side of the bed until I was sitting upright with my feet planted on the floor. Mary stirred in the dark. Two months earlier, moving to an upright position so quickly would have set my head spinning. I would have spent several seconds in a daze, trying to figure out where I was and what I was supposed to do next. But that was two months ago.

Now, in the first week of August 2003, I was instantly awake and alert. The dimly glowing numbers on the alarm clock indicated it was almost 4:30 am. Time to get up. I went to my closet and dressed quickly—gym shorts, a light shirt, athletic socks and running shoes, was all I needed. Muffled footsteps followed by a sliver of light that peeked beneath my closet door announced Mary's intention to join me.

I went downstairs and waited. Mary followed soon after. I retrieved a house key and we both stepped quietly through the darkened lower level of our house to the front door. The street was deserted, but we could hear a chorus of night creatures: frogs, bats, crickets, and one insomniac dog, barking somewhere in the dark.

A Life Unburdened

. . . .

Mary and I walked quietly down the driveway to the street. "Look at these slackers," I said, glancing around at the darkened homes of my neighbors who had the good sense to remain in bed at such an early hour. Mary smiled politely at the tired joke. I had said it every morning for the last two months. We turned south and began the one-mile loop around our neighborhood. The route includes a steep hill that always left me huffing heavily by the time I reached the top. We would walk this route five times on this morning, for more than an hour. It would be the fourth time this week.

This had been our morning ritual for the last few weeks. Up at 4:15 am, out by 4:30 am. We had a hard time describing exactly what it was we had been doing for the last two months. We didn't like the word "diet" because it was an inadequate description of the change we had experienced. This was no diet, no temporary adjustment of what we were eating so we could lose a few pounds. We were literally trying to remake ourselves—physically, mentally, emotionally, intellectually, and spiritually.

When we started in June, I was unable to do much walking. My back and legs hurt and my hands and feet would swell up uncomfortably, so initially we just changed our diet. I felt better immediately, but for the first two months or so, I saw little weight loss, although my clothes got looser.

These early morning walks began as simple exercise, but evolved over time into our mobile office, psychiatrist's couch and relationship counseling sessions. Like any couple who has been married for 17 years, there was much that went unsaid between us. When you walk in circles in the dark for an hour, then two hours, you've got to do something to fill the time, so we talked about life, love, regrets and joys, anger and forgiveness, politics and prose, death and resurrection, our plans, our aspirations and our fears. We talked about anything and everything. It eventually dawned on us that we were getting up early in the morning, not to walk, but to enjoy each other's company, discuss the day ahead, plan for our future, laugh, get angry with each other and simply communicate. Not only did we grow slimmer after more than one year of walking, we also grew closer. Later, as we grew healthier and were able to see a future for ourselves that transcended the confining roles defined by an over-commercialized society, we exercised our entrepreneurial muscles and worked up the courage to pursue business opportunities we had only dreamed of before. Our morning walks, which previously had revolved around our personal lives, now doubled as business meetings. Our one mile course became our new conference room.

It wasn't always easy. Sometimes we would finish a walk in silence, allowing for a bruised ego or an aching heart to heal. Other times, we laughed over some nearly forgotten incident until tears welled in our eyes. Most times though, our walks were a joyous celebration of the new future we envisioned together—a future without the discomfort of poor health. I was amazed at how, after nearly 20 years together, so much had been left unsaid between us and so much was left to say.

Our daughters slept during these early morning expeditions, but by the time they awoke, the house was filled with the aroma of breakfast. On most days, breakfast included eggs—real eggs, not the anemic egg whites that I subsisted on during my low-fat days. The eggs were often accompanied by nitrite-free bacon or done up as an omelet with vegetables and meat left over from yesterday's dinner. Sometimes we had un-homogenized whole milk with our breakfast.

MORE CHANGES

Besides our early morning walks, the most obvious change in our household was the food we ate. Gone were the frozen bags of pre-cooked chicken parts from the bulk foods warehouse. The thick slabs of frozen heat-and-serve toast that we used to eat were missing too, and there were no more empty bags of chips, bottles of soda, or take-out pizza boxes to gather up for the weekly trash collection. The drive-thru cashiers at several of the fast food outlets I frequented were, no doubt, concerned over my absence, as I am certain I contributed significantly toward their monthly revenue goals.

We did most of our shopping at the local farmers' market and at stores that specialized in whole foods products. We tried to stick to the basics: meat, seafood, fruits, vegetables and dairy products. Of course, our parting of the ways with processed food could best be described as a separation rather than a full-fledged divorce. At the time, I still believed that soy was a healthy food for me and continued to purchase tofu products. I was not yet completely immune to the lure of junk food either.

THE LOW POINT

One day, after work, I had to stop for gas. I was hungry and wanted something to eat for the long ninety-minute commute home. I surveyed the gas station store aisles and found nothing but snack food. I don't even remember what my excuse was, but somehow, I rationalized the purchase of a family-sized bag of potato chips as a "healthy" alternative to the rest of the fare available. I gassed up and kept one eye on the interstate while I struggled to open the bag of chips with one hand.

There's an old movie, *The Days of Wine and Roses*, which stars Jack Lemon as an alcoholic struggling to overcome his demons. In one riveting scene, Jack's character attempts to rehabilitate himself by spending time with his father-in-law, helping out with the family's garden business. Jack had hidden a bottle of liquor in one of the potted plants in the greenhouse and had planned to sneak in at night and drink it while everyone else was sleep. Unfortunately, he forgot which planter he hid the bottle in. What started as a simple recovery operation turned into a manic search-and-destroy mission instead. By the time he found the bottle, he had completely destroyed the greenhouse. He got drunk nevertheless, which only made him feel worse.

As I plowed into that bag of greasy, salty, artificially flavored potato chips, I was the drunk in *The Days of Wine and Roses*. I told myself, "I'll only eat a few," just enough to take the edge off my hunger, but I knew I would not—could not—stop. When it was over, I crumpled up the empty bag with my greasy, free hand and flung it to the floor of the car in disgust. I had managed to stay "clean" for several weeks, and now this. What's worse, my hunger had not abated. I just felt sick, physically and emotionally. It was then that I saw so clearly the control that unhealthy food had over me. It made me angry at myself and at the nameless, faceless corporate entity that made access to these foods so easy and inviting—like the friendly neighborhood drug dealer who always has just what you think you need. That was my low point. I would never reach that point again.

FOOD TRACKER

Early hunter-gatherer societies had to become quite skilled at tracking their food if they wanted to eat. In September of 2003, I too learned to track my food. I acquired a new weapon in my arsenal of weight loss gadgets, a software program called "Diet and Exercise." I installed it on the Palm handheld that I took with me everywhere. This program enabled me to accurately track the food I ate, along with the number of calories and the macronutrient breakdown. Previously, I had kept a written account, noting every morsel that passed my lips. At the end of the day, I entered this data into a spreadsheet. It was a cumbersome but effective way to track my food intake.

The electronic tracker was wonderful because it had a huge database of foods and enabled me to run "what-if" scenarios. If I was trying to stick to a set number of calories on a given day, I could plug in different meal options to determine how much of a particular food item I could have without exceeding my calorie count. My daily calories averaged around 2000. This was important, because as someone who had paid little attention to how much I ate for the past ten years, I needed to relearn how to control my portions. Doing so helped teach my body to adjust to fewer calories. It must be noted that it was only through eating whole satisfying foods that I was able to control portions.

A Life Unburdened

Another benefit of food tracking was that when I reviewed what I had eaten over the course of a month, I could see patterns in my eating behavior that I might not otherwise have noticed. I saw, for instance, that I ate more on Saturdays than any other day of the week. I also noted that when I tried to cut my calories below what was a normal amount for me (about 2000), I could only maintain this reduced-calorie level for two or three days. After that, my records typically revealed a sudden spike in food intake, a binge, usually on the third or fourth day. I could also see connections between food intake and mood. If I was stuck in traffic on the way home, there was usually a spike in calorie consumption soon afterward. This information was very helpful because it made me more aware, not just of what I was eating, but when I was eating and why. Thus, having identified harmful behavior patterns, I was able to work toward changing them.

I was sold on the value of food tracking, but Mary hated it. Attending to the minutia of tracking ran counter to the more freestyle approach she took to cooking and eating. She had far more control than I over her eating behavior and did not need the extra help that tracking provides. Inevitably, we locked horns over the issue. A typical pre-dinner conversation went something like this:

"Mmmm, that smells good. Are we having chili?" I'd ask.

"Yes," would come her clipped reply, along with a sudden drop in temperature in the room.

I'd start with a little small talk and work toward my real point of interest. "I didn't eat much for lunch and traffic was pretty bad today. I've really been looking forward to dinner." I'd pause to gauge her response, and then continue. "Hey are those jalapeño peppers I smell? Oh yeah, you're making it spicy the way I like it—so what else is in there?" This was the moment of truth.

She would take a deep breath, set her jaw, then list the ingredients without taking her eyes off the stove or stopping what she was doing. "Hamburger, peppers, onions, tomatoes. . . ." The list continued until she was finished and then silence.

Chapter Nine: The Road Home

. . . .

"So how much hamburger did you put in?"

A long silence. When she cooked, Mary made due with whatever ingredients were available—a pinch here, a smidgen there—that was her style. As mother, home school teacher, primary cook, soccer practice chauffeur, household accountant and hair braider, she found food and ingredient tracking an unnecessary complication to her already busy life.

Her reply usually came in the form of a rough estimate which I generally regarded as an inadequate reply to my excruciating demand for exactness. These opening shots served as a preamble to an undeclared cold war expressed through exasperated sighs, cold shoulders, steely glares and stony silence. Thankfully, this was the only issue we ever clashed over as we worked toward remaking our lives.

THE HOLIDAYS: A DIETER'S NIGHTMARE

By October of 2003, I was feeling like a new man. Four months of healthier eating and exercise had worked a miracle. I was tracking my weight and was overjoyed to see that for several weeks, I had lost almost six pounds per week. My clothes were falling off me and my energy was up. I no longer minded going walking at 4:30 am. In fact, I looked forward to it. Along with rising early, I had finally adjusted to going to bed at nine o'clock at night. Giving up late night TV was the only way to ensure I could get enough sleep to keep such early morning hours. Although my weight still hovered north of 300 pounds, I had lost somewhere around fifty pounds or more and I felt great. My goal for the year end was to break the 300-pound barrier by Christmas.

Anyone who has ever tried to lose weight knows that the holidays are a treacherous time of the year. From about mid-October through the end of December, food becomes a principal component of every thought, conversation and action. It starts with Halloween candy, complete with orange and black sugary confections, candied apples and those Styrofoam-like peanut candies.

A Life Unburdened

. . . .

Next comes the Mount Everest of food holidays: Thanksgiving. When I was growing up, the days leading up to turkey day turned my every-day world into a mythical land of candied ham, sweet potato pies, banana pudding, spicy dressing with succulent chunks of meat and crunchy celery, potato salad with sweet nuggets of apples, oven baked rolls smothered in butter, cornbread and collard greens, sweet onions, cranberry sauce and homemade ice cream.

Finally, Christmas. Another turkey, ham or both. Cookies, cheese and caramel popcorn, more pies, hard candies, mounds of salted mixed nuts, sweet apples, oranges and tangerines and a cake or two. Even though in my adult years the amount of holiday food we ate had been scaled back dramatically, it was still the food season as far as I was concerned.

At Christmas, the strong are separated from the weak. In the old days, we would have given in to the temptations of the holidays, packing in more food and packing on more weight, but not this time. Our mostly whole foods diet had an unexpected effect on us. Whenever we attempted to lose weight in the past, it was always a struggle. We were always shadowed by cravings for the sticky-sweet salty foods we loved, so we were a bit surprised to find that those cravings had evaporated.

This was a revelation. We were beginning to understand that our carbohydrate-rich, nutrient-poor, processed food diet actually made us want to eat more, sparking cravings for certain foods that always defeated us in the end. We decided not to buy any Halloween candy, but Thanksgiving and Christmas turned out to be quite a surprise when we discovered on December 31st, 2003 that we actually lost weight over the holidays. I did not cross the 300-pound barrier as I had hoped, but I was much closer.

THE WESTON A. PRICE FOUNDATION

It was in December that I discovered the Weston A. Price Foundation, an organization dedicated to the research of Dr. Price and which educates consumers about the value of whole food traditional diets, and helps them find these foods.

Dr. Price's work and that of the Foundation affected me deeply in part because it made so much sense and answered a lot of questions. The chief message of the Foundation was that food had to provide liberal amounts of the nutrients the body needs—not the minimal Recommended Daily Allowances, but liberal amounts. Otherwise physical degeneration would occur, with each generation becoming less fit than the previous one.

Finally, here was a plausible explanation for why the health of my family seemed to be declining with each succeeding generation. I could see now why, despite my best efforts to exercise and eat right, I still managed to slowly gain weight. Here then was an explanation for why I saw so many more overweight grade-school-aged kids. I was beginning to see why exercise never seemed to provide the return on investment that I thought it should. It was becoming clear to me just how critical a role food played in my health. I never believed the argument popular with sectors of the food industry and many health officials that it didn't matter what I ate so long as I exercised. I didn't believe the subtle message from many of the experts that obesity is simply the result of laziness and a conscious choice to overeat. I knew I wasn't lazy, and I knew that I never chose to be fat. I knew that some foods did make me feel lazy sometimes while other foods left me feeling energized. The idea, promoted by the diet professionals, that all food is the same, just didn't match my experience.

Also, it didn't make sense to me that the definition of good health seemed to revolve around body weight and nothing else. I knew a number of people, such as diabetics, who were very thin, but being thin didn't make them healthy. But this was the message I had been hearing for most of my life: health equals thin and thin equals a low-fat diet. It seemed to me that nutrition leaders and industry interests had engaged in a calculated effort to avoid discussion of the nutritive quality of our food and focus only on caloric quantity. And since fats have twice the calories as protein or carbohydrates, these experts argued that the ticket to good health was a scale-back of fat to the bare minimum—no egg yolks, no cream, no fat on your meat, no lard and no butter. Yet Weston Price discovered that these fats carried the most important vitamins of all.

When I was a kid, no one counted calories. We simply ate the food that was available. A lot of this food—full-fat dairy products and red meat—are the very foods that I had been warned to avoid for most of my adult life. How was it possible, then, that once people became more conscious of diet and weight, started counting calories and eating diet food, the percentage of overweight and obese people actually increased?

Something was seriously wrong with what I came to see as the Fat Hypothesis. It seemed the low-fat, high-carbohydrate processed food prescription for preventing obesity and heart disease was actually causing these epidemics.

The other reason the work of Dr. Price and the Foundation struck a chord with me is that so much of what they taught sounded like advice from my mother. She never badgered me to go outside and get exercise, she didn't have to. I was a pretty active kid. She did, however, spend a lot of time extolling the healthful virtues of traditional foods. She would have been appalled at my consumption of simulated soy foods, breakfast pastries, margarine and fast food. For most of my childhood, she always kept a garden in our backyard. She believed in the concept of organic produce long before the idea became mainstream. She purchased a side of beef once and in the good times always kept our horizontal freezer well stocked with everything from fillet mignon to stew bones. She knew how to render lard from fatback and understood the nutritive value of soup made from fish heads. She plied me with chicken soup and bone broth when I was ill, and cod liver oil to keep me well. She believed in cooking from scratch and rarely bought food pre-cooked. She was wary of food additives and was a voracious consumer of books on health.

And yet, despite her commitment to good health, she was not immune to the seductive temptation of affordable convenience foods. For a time, she strayed from her roots, but eventually returned to the food she knew best.

At the age of 43 years I discovered what most of us discover eventually. Mom was right all along.

THERE'S NO PLACE LIKE HOME, FOR EXERCISE

In September we decided, as an early Christmas gift, to convert an unfinished room in our basement into a home gym. We already had a flat weight bench, a rowing machine and an older treadmill, but the problem was that this equipment was crowded into a small space. There wasn't really enough room for everything, so we kept the treadmill folded up and moved the rowing machine from its storage space when we wanted to use it.

The lack of space often gave me an excuse not to exercise, so when we decided to turn the spare room into a gym, it seemed like the perfect solution.

First we brought in workmen to hang the drywall and paint. We then took over from there. I laid down a padded floor made of interlocking puzzle-like pieces of dense black foam, then ran a four-inch black strip around the entire room to create the effect of a baseboard. Next we hung three large mirrors along one wall, transforming the once-drab room into something that looked like a gym. Last, we brought in the equipment which included the treadmill, the flat bench, a set of dumbbells and a barbell bench with stations for bench pressing, butterflies, leg presses, preacher curls. We also put in a stationary bike, and later, a new treadmill, an elliptical machine and a heavy bag for boxing. As a finishing touch, I added a black locker where we stored our weight-lifting equipment, boxing gloves and towels. A large industrial fan and a CD stereo system completed the furnishings. It was good, but the walls were too bare, so I added a white board for writing out the day's exercise routine and added a stainless steel peg board for posting pictures or notes on the wall. We decided not to install a television as we thought it might provide too much of a distraction and a temptation to return to our old ways.

When I walked into the gym and closed the door, an amazing thing happened. Suddenly, I wasn't at home anymore. I was at the gym. I found that by creating a total exercise immersion environment, I was motivated to do just that. I realize a home gym isn't an option for everyone, but when I consider what a difference it has made in my life, I will never be without one again. For me, spare bedrooms, game rooms and home theatres all take a back seat in priority to a home gym.

I enjoy exercising as it has made a big difference in my life, but I still believe that exercise has been oversold as a cure-all for everything. Why, for instance, is it so difficult to stick to a routine? Why does something that is supposed to be so healthy hurt so much? Like many things in life, exercise has two faces. The right amount of sensible exercise, supported with good nutrition, can be a boon to your health. Too much of the wrong exercise on the wrong diet can do the opposite. Let's take a look at the myth of exercise and explore ways to make exercise work for you.

Chapter Ten

What You Don't Know About Exercise

Why exercise alone won't solve your health problems

The new dietary guidelines for Americans recommends that those adults hoping to sustain weight loss should engage in 60 to 90 minutes of moderate intensity exercise each day. The diet doctors never tire of reminding us that the key to weight loss is simple: eat less, exercise more. Some experts will go so far as to suggest that what you eat is irrelevant, as long as you maintain a caloric expenditure that exceeds your caloric intake. Exercise has been touted as a cure-all for many ailments. With all of the hyperbole surrounding the benefits of regular exercise, it's easy to see why many people view it as the magic bullet that can solve all of their problems.

There's little doubt that great benefits derive from exercise. Our bodies were designed to be challenged physically. Our muscles revel in the task of straining against opposing forces; running, swimming and sports exhilarate us. Our exquisitely designed cardiovascular system hums merrily along when our demand for blood and oxygen increases through aerobic workouts. And let us not forget the psychological and emotional benefits derived from physical work as well.

Once, when I worked as a software developer, my coworkers and I decided to rearrange our office space by reconfiguring the layout of our cubicles. The individual slabs that made up the cubicle walls were old and quite heavy, having been manufactured sometime around the 1970s.

As software developers, we normally spent our days comfortably settled in front of a computer. On this day however, we took turns grunting, sweating, and cursing as we dragged the huge slabs of cloth-covered metal, from one end of the office to the other. Despite the difficulty of the work, the pinched fingers and stubbed toes, I recall feeling elated by the end of the day. It wasn't just the sense of euphoria one experiences from physical labor, it was also the sense of accomplishment and the feeling that I had actually completed something important, a rare experience in the software world. I left work that day feeling like a new man, albeit a sweaty and disheveled one.

So what's wrong with exercise? Nothing really. The problem is that exercise has been grossly oversold as a cure-all for weight loss and health maintenance. Take the new guidelines for example. If you're overweight, it is very likely that you're also out of shape. Exercising for 60 to 90 minutes per day is a noble goal, but it may not realistically be possible for you in your condition. If the only way for you to lose weight is by exercising for an hour and a half each day, you're stuck in a catch-22 scenario. This is a perfect example of weight loss theory colliding with weight gain reality. The myth of exercise is that exercise alone provides the answer to losing weight, maintaining weight loss, and sustaining a high level of fitness.

Anyone who has ever started the New Year by joining a gym and spending the next two weeks working feverishly to get in shape eventually experiences the down-side of exercise. After punishing the body for days on end, you invariably fall ill from overexertion or wind up injuring yourself.

Of course, you could always take it slow by adopting the familiar "small steps" approach which we've heard so much about recently. Small steps may work for someone who is relatively fit already, but for those of us who have passed the point of no return, small steps simply won't work for the same reason that trying to fill an empty swimming pool one teacup at a time won't work. While it is technically feasible, it's not very likely to result in success. The small-steps approach to weight loss suffers from the assumption that you can solve a big problem with little effort, and change your behavior toward exercise without changing anything else in your life. It is simply not realistic to think that walking a few extra steps per day is sufficient to counter the damage wrought by years of inactivity and a diet that consists of bagels and donuts for breakfast, salads, burgers and fries for lunch, and a bucket of spaghetti and meatballs for dinner. Real success in weight loss and health gains comes from developing a strategic multidisciplinary plan that incorporates the following steps:

- A willingness to educate yourself about how your body works
- A willingness to make a lifelong commitment toward your goals
- Soliciting support from family, friends and professionals
- Creating harmony in your life by identifying areas of stress and working toward solutions to reduce that stress
- Cutting through the hype of our over-commercialized consumer society and learning to identify what really is important in life
- Adopting an improved approach to what you eat, with an emphasis on real foods
- Developing and implementing a realistic exercise program
- Getting high-quality sleep
- Applying your newfound sense of empowerment toward achieving personal goals
- Sharing what you've learned with others

I have found that an effort that includes anything less than what I've listed above is likely doomed to failure. It may be possible to lose weight and appear healthy, through sheer willpower and an above average tolerance for pain. Over time, though, our bodies will simply break down under the twin burdens of too much exercise and too little nutrition. Take a look at marathon runners toward the end of the pack as they cross the finish line. These are high performance athletes, yet exercise can turn them into stumbling corpses. What do you think it will do for you with your new year's gym membership and six years of inactivity to your credit?

Many weight loss plans call for restricted calories based on low-fat, low-energy foods. This is the reduced-calorie side of the diet equation. Imagine eating lots of fiber-rich salad, a sliver of skinless chicken breast and drinking lots of water. Full? Of course you are. Satisfied? Not likely. Now go exercise. According to some of the most popular weight loss plans, you're now expected to go out and engage in moderate intensity exercise for 60 to 90 minutes, and you're expected to do this over and over again. Good luck.

Do we really believe the Great Plains Indians of the 1800s were fueling up on salads before engaging in the demanding labor of running down buffalo? Were the Inuit of Alaska topping off their tanks with low-fat meal replacement shakes before heading out across the ice to track seal?

When I tried to exercise and follow a low-fat diet plan, I found I often grew tired long before an hour was up. Very often, by the last 15 minutes of exercise, my workouts looked like the thrashings of a dying man since I had used up most of the "energy" from my meager diet in the first 15 to 20 minutes. I usually felt like a failure at the end of one of these exercise sessions. Imagine having a full stomach, but still feeling hungry, and now, because of a poor workout, add mild depression to this stew of troubles. Try repeating this scenario over the course of a couple weeks. It's easy to see why people simply give up, order an extra large pizza and plant themselves in front of the TV. The idea that you can consume less energy at the table, but somehow expend more energy in the gym is ridiculous. While it is true that burning more calories than you consume will result in weight loss, this premise is only true if you've consumed enough of the right kind of energy to fuel both your body and your mind. Failing this, your workouts may only serve to remind you of how miserable you are. The high failure rate that many of us experience when it comes to dieting and exercise suggests that low-energy eating coupled with attempts at high-energy exercise fail far more often than they succeed. Yet many experts swear by this method. When failure inevitably comes, the problem is never due to the flawed method, but with your apparent lack of willpower.

One of the latest trends in exercise is the 10,000 steps fad. Pedometers have been flying off the shelves as people try to meet the new dietary guidelines by walking 10,000 steps per day. This is a noble cause to be sure, but if you're overweight and in poor physical condition, walking 10,000 steps everyday is virtually impossible.

When I weighed over 400 pounds, walking even 100 steps was difficult. I found that no amount of willpower could overcome a knee that slips out of place and a lower back that grinds with pain after only five minutes of walking. Consuming a low-energy, high-carbohydrate diet based on highly processed foods, grains, salads and vegetable oils, and then trying to exercise for 30 minutes, let alone 60 to 90, was simply out of the question. My diet at the time left me listless, unsatisfied, fatigued and despondent. Even if I had somehow possessed the physical energy to exercise, I still would have lacked the mental desire to do so. Why, then, has the government devised new dietary and fitness recommendations which, for people like me, are practically guaranteed to fail?

Yet the new dietary guidelines put much more emphasis on physical activity than the previous ones. Why such a focus on exercise? The food lobby is very powerful. No one in that industry wants to see restrictions put on the foods that yield the highest profits, namely most of the products on your grocer's shelf, products composed of cheap ingredients—starch, sugar, MSG, trans fats and soy—in other words, processed convenience foods. The reason the dietary guidelines put so much focus on exercise is that it allows the creators of the guidelines to avoid the politically sensitive issue of food. The focus on exercise avoids the unpleasant task of telling the truth about the food we eat and setting meaningful restrictions on the types of food we consume.

A Life Unburdened

....

How else can we justify dietary advice that says "there's no such thing as bad food," that tells us the quantity of food—the amount of calories—is what's really important, not quality. In other words, it's OK to eat pretty much anything so long as you count calories. By this reasoning, a diet of soda, glazed donuts and potato chips is acceptable, if you don't eat too much and get plenty of exercise. This "anything goes" approach is good news for the food industry, but bad news for the rest of us. By putting the focus on exercise, the food industry is absolved of any responsibility for the nation's growing weight problem.

Of course, some of the blame falls on ourselves as we have become a woefully sedentary people, and we have stubbornly refused to educate ourselves about how our bodies work and what we should eat. But the sharing of responsibility is the foundation of a civilized society. Where, then, is the social responsibility of an industry that makes unsubstantiated health claims about products, promotes fattening foods for dieters, cloaks harmful additives like MSG under consumer-friendly names like "flavors," and preys on children with empty treats designed to heighten their sensitivity to the very foods that contribute most to poor health?

Where is the social responsibility of our elected officials whom we have entrusted to protect us from a predatory free market system that puts corporate profit above personal health? Finally, where is the social responsibility of our prescription-drug-addicted medical community? Why have they wasted decades obsessing over dietary animal fat when they knew, or should have known, that it was the trans fats found in partially hydrogenated vegetable oils, snack foods and baked goods that were harming us—that excessive sugars, starches and additives in America's diet of ready-to-eat convenience foods were the principal destroyers of our health?

One final myth about exercise is the idea that you can form a new exercise habit in just six months. Occasionally this happens, but not often. Just look at the failure rate of most diets and exercise routines. In many cases, we never make it to the six-month mark. Rarely does exercise become a lifelong habit. I found that after a year of vegetarianism, and on another diet, after at least six months of regular trips to the gym, quitting was effortlessly easy. I believe my failure in both cases had everything to do with an inadequate diet. When I finally improved my diet in the summer of 2003, maintaining a routine of regular exercise suddenly became possible. Habits, for the most part, can only be formed when we derive some pleasure from the activity in question. Because I found little pleasure in vegetarianism and spending long hours in a commercial gym, those activities never became habits. If you are currently on a diet or participating in an exercise program from which you derive little joy, your chance of lasting success is nil.

THE TRUTH ABOUT EXERCISE

So what's the truth about exercise? Exercise is essential for weight loss and health maintenance, but exercise is only one strategy in a multi-part approach to better health. Before you put on your walking shoes, be aware that without a proper diet that limits or eliminates some foods, while including or increasing the consumption of others, you're only addressing one part of the problem. Before you assume you know which foods are bad for your health and preventing you from getting the full benefit of exercise, make sure you've read the chapters in Section 4 and reviewed the resources section. It's also important to reduce stress in your life. Getting plenty of sleep on a regular basis is another factor that helped us achieve success in our efforts to lose weight.

WHY IS EXERCISE SO DIFFICULT?

Even with a good diet, reduced stress and plenty of sleep, you may still find regular exercise difficult to sustain. Historically speaking, exercise—that is, the act of engaging in a physically demanding activity for the sole purpose of maintaining physical fitness—is a relatively new concept. Our hunter-gatherer ancestors and their agrarian descendents had little need for exercise. Why would they, given the physically demanding lives they led? Except for professional athletes and others whose work is physically demanding, most of us can manage our daily lives with very little exercise. This is a markedly different situation compared to our ancestors, whose very survival required them to be physically active.

If you were to propose to a homesteader of the 1890s that he should get up in the morning and go to a place where he could run on a treadmill and lift heavy objects, he would think you mad. He would wonder why anyone would waste all that energy running in place and working up a sweat when it could more fruitfully be applied to mending fences, building a barn or hunting for food. The lives we lived were once in balance with our bodies' requirements for optimal health. In our modern lives today, where much of the physical labor has been eliminated, we have fallen out of balance with activity needs.

In my early career as a graphic designer, I often worked at a large drafting table standing up. In the days before computers, I used the familiar tools of the draftsman—the T-square, triangle and ruler. My work required a fair amount of reaching, bending and squatting. In those days, my profession required moving about the office and around the company where I worked. I often spent up to half my day on my feet. Today, I sit in an office in front of a computer. With a telephone, computer, the Internet and email, I can conduct my entire business from the comfort of my desk. The price I and many others have paid for this "progress" is chronic inactivity and compromised health.

To compensate, we exercise, which is little more than an artificial copy of the real work we used to do. The problem is that while our bodies are designed to handle physical challenge, as humans our brains are hardwired to work only when there is a clear purpose for the work. Without the clear purpose of building shelter, defending our family or finding food, physical exercise seems pointless. This is why walking on a treadmill is literally a nonproductive activity since even the dullest toddler knows that the purpose of walking is to get from point A to point B. If a man is required to walk five miles each day to tend his flock, he does so because there is a clear purpose in the effort directly connected to his own survival. If the same man attempts to walk on a treadmill for five miles every day, the effort seems rather pointless, even when his doctor insists he needs to exercise to protect his heart.

For most of us, no amount of scaremongering about premature death from heart disease, diabetes and stroke is enough to motivate us to exercise regularly. It is only when we have had a close call with the reaper that we finally see the relevant connection to exercise, but even a brush with death loses its sting after a sufficient amount of time has passed, and the football-and-spicy-nachos season rolls around again.

The challenge is how to make exercise relevant enough in our lives so that we are motivated to do it on a regular basis? Most of us live in densely packed housing in the city or the suburbs, so wandering out to tend our flock on a daily basis is not an option. If you are fortunate enough to live in a pedestrian friendly area where walking is feasible, you can leave the car in the garage and walk to the store, the bus stop or even the office. Parking further from the entrance to your place of business and taking the stairs are two "small steps" that you can do, but realistically, they may contribute very little to your overall health unless your company has a parking lot the size of Delaware. There's always the option of chucking your modern life, selling your home in the suburbs and moving out to the country on a few acres in an attempt to create the kind of lifestyle more conducive to good health. For some people this really is an option, but for most of us it isn't. What are we to do then?

WHAT WE DID

Mary and I realized that we couldn't make all of the exercise we would need to do relevant beyond just exercise, but we did discover several ways to make exercise more meaningful. In addition to our morning walks, we added bicycling. We found that riding a bike the 10 miles or so to the farmers' market became a highly relevant activity, connected with procuring food. We live on a half-acre parcel with a large swath of unruly lawn. At least twice a month, Mary pushes a lawn mower up and down the hill at the back of the lot, achieving a workout that rivals anything she can do in the gym.

When we put in a raised-bed garden, we had to purchase fill dirt to fill the two garden boxes we built. More than a half ton of dirt was hauled to our home by the supplier and dumped in the street—more than 30 yards from the garden. We spent the entire day hauling wheelbarrow loads of dirt from the street to the garden. When the boxes were filled, we had to haul the extra dirt an additional 10 yards up the steep hill behind our house. It was backbreaking work that left us exhausted and exhilarated. These alternate exercise activities were not random "small steps," but were part of a larger plan to add more physical activity to our daily lives.

Everything from turning the earth in our garden to trimming trees and cleaning out the garage became a meaningful opportunity to exercise. If you examine your life closely, you can probably find ways to make exercise more meaningful, too. Of course, once you learn to make some exercises more practical, you may discover the impractical ones, like walking on a treadmill, are easier and more enjoyable.

We also exercised in our gym. We needed a few weeks with our new eating plan before we had the mental and physical energy to begin our program. And build us up it did. I was actually quite surprised at how much better I felt after only a few weeks away from most of the convenience foods we used to eat.

When we did begin to exercise, I decided that it would be useful for us to keep track of what exercises we did and how often we did them. I drew up a check sheet on the computer that listed several exercises, like walking and weight-lifting routines. I included a row that showed the dates for the month and a column for checking off which days I exercised and which exercise I did on each day. I printed out this chart and stuck it up on the wall in the gym.

We set a goal of a minimum of five days per week for exercise, alternating aerobic exercise (walking, jogging and the treadmill) with anaerobic exercise like weight lifting.

Chapter Ten: What You Don't Know About Exercise

· ·

One final point regarding exercise: do not fall victim to the myth of the perfect body. For women, this means that you should not feel compelled to transform yourself into a life-sized Barbie doll. Men, don't stress over the fact that you don't have washboard abs. These messages are part of a consumer engineering effort designed to make us feel bad about ourselves so we'll continue to buy products and services that will supposedly make us happier. They won't. It is enough to love the body you have, whatever its imperfections.

THE TOOLS WE USE: FITNESS TRACKERS

I was no stranger to exercise, but when I decided to make a change for the better, I knew I needed something other than just a fuzzy idea in my head about my workout program. I needed a real plan and a way to track my progress. Why track? Early on, I was feeling a bit frustrated because, like many people, I wanted to see instant results. Two months after I began my exercise program I didn't see much progress. I was working out almost every day I thought—or was I? I checked my tracker, which was a simple printed spreadsheet with a list of exercises, dates and a checkbox to denote when I exercised. I discovered that on most weeks I was working out only three days a week. That wasn't how I remembered it of course, but my tracker told the truth.

I also created a spreadsheet for weight training exercises with space for dates, sets and reps. I found lots of professionally produced video clips on the internet that demonstrated how to do the exercises properly. Whenever I worked out, I simply checked off that day. I found it helpful to alternate exercises so as not to overwork any particular body part, and to alternate workout days and factor in an occasional day off.

BODY FAT ANALYZER

Your body fat is the ratio of fat to lean body mass (muscle). A quick check on the internet will turn up a body fat chart that shows what your body fat should allegedly be for your weight and height. I don't consider these charts to be the definitive word on what my body fat ratio should be. Remember, one-size-fits-all solutions rarely work, but they can provide a helpful guide.

There are a number of ways to measure your body fat. I use an impedance device, an electronic device with metal sensors that send a low-level electrical signal through your body. No, it doesn't hurt. The lean tissue in your body has a higher percentage of water, and so conducts the signal more quickly than does the fat in your body. The device then calculates your body fat with this data.

So how accurate is this method? I don't know. Depending upon the device used, when you do the measurement, and whether you've had any water, you can get different results. So why use it? When I was a vegetarian, I lost about fifty pounds, but found I was weak and tired easily. I suspect that along with the fat, I lost quite a bit of muscle mass as well. Measuring my body fat, even if the measurement is inaccurate, is useful for showing whether I'm losing fat or gaining muscle mass over time. I perform the measurement at the same time of day under the same conditions so the results are consistent, if not entirely accurate. I found this to be a useful tool for tracking progress early.

Mary doesn't share my obsession with technology and my penchant for gathering arcane bits of data, and so does not bother checking her body fat. "I can see all the body fat I want in a mirror, thank you," is her characteristic reply.

BATHROOM SCALES

Some of you may be afraid of the scale. I know I was. Get over it. It's not like people haven't noticed that you have a weight problem. The irony is that the only person you're keeping this "secret" from is you. It's natural to want to avoid bad news, but avoiding a problem prevents you from solving it, so get thee to a scale and face the fat. Can't find a scale at the local discount-mart that goes up high enough? You may need to order one. I've seen scales that go close to 400 pounds. I've read about scales that go higher.

· ·

My scale is an analog scale, the kind with the red needle. Personally I don't trust the electronic ones since, if I stood on my laptop, I wouldn't expect it to work properly either. This is my own personal bias, as I've heard there's not much difference between an electronic and an analog scale.

Use the scale, but do not live and die by it. One of the unsolved mysteries of weight loss is the fact that you can drop clothing sizes, look slimmer in the mirror, and elicit lustful stares from strangers, yet still weigh the same for many weeks in a row. The explanation typically offered is that you're gaining muscle as you're losing fat, and that's how you're able to get physically smaller but weigh the same. I don't completely buy this argument, as it would have to be some kind of coincidence for you to gain in muscle the exact amount of fat lost, and unless you're a high-performance athlete, don't expect to gain a lot of muscle anyway. Use the scale as just one measure of your success, a guide, nothing more. How often you weigh yourself is up to you: once a week, once a day, or once a month, it's your call.

TAPE MEASURE

Bathroom scales can be frustrating when they fail to register obvious progress evidenced by your clothes, mood and envious friends. A tape measure may be just the ticket for helping you see your success. Common body parts to measure are the waist, hips, thigh, chest, neck, and calf.

For some people, finding your waist may represent a challenge. Unfortunately, fitness experts can't seem to agree on where exactly the waist is. Some say above the navel. Some say below the navel. Others say just below the rib cage, or the thinnest section of your lower trunk. What do you do if there is no "thinnest" section of your trunk or your rib cage has gone missing? I shoot for the area between the navel and the rib cage. Close enough, I think.

. . . .

BLOOD PRESSURE GAUGE

If you're overweight, there's a good chance that your blood pressure may be higher than what is recommended for healthy individuals. There are different schools of thought on what this means. Some medical experts believe that hypertension is a precursor to heart disease while others believe that heart disease comes first, and that high blood pressure is symptomatic of an ill heart. Confused? Here's more to baffle you: the numbers that constitute high blood pressure have been revised downward over the years. Where 120/80 used to be considered a normal blood pressure, this number has recently been redefined as pre-hypertensive. Some pessimists suggest that this change in the guidelines has little to do with concern for our health and everything to do with expanding the market for expensive blood pressure medications. I tend to agree. Whatever side of the argument you fall on, you should research the whole story on blood pressure, then make your own decisions. Exercise, a good diet and weight loss have been shown to improve blood pressure, just remember that blood pressure goes up naturally and gradually with age (the old standard was your age plus 100 over 90). Some people can even go off their medication by controlling their blood pressure through lifestyle changes. We did.

FITNESS EQUIPMENT FOR THE GYM

A home gym isn't for everyone, but if you have the room, it is one of the best investments you can make on behalf of yourself and your family.

A set of dumbbells and a weight bench is one of the cheapest, most versatile and most effective investments you can make. There are literally hundreds of exercises you can do with just dumbbells and a bench (an incline bench is even better). It goes without saying that heavy objects made of iron can be dangerous when used improperly. Study up first, start slow and be safe.

I also recommend a barbell bench that allows for bench presses, preacher curls, leg lifts, etc. When I'm walking outside, I sometimes use a weight vest and ankle weights. Walking with weights can be a good low-impact way to increase the intensity of your walks. Weight vests can be adjusted from 0 up to their maximum weight and can feel quite heavy when you first try one on. If you use a vest, make sure you're already in fairly good shape. Start small, real small, with very light weights (5 – 10 pounds). Go slow, be safe.

Even though I am a big proponent of home gyms, commercial gyms can still be a very valuable component in your exercise plan. In fact, from time to time, I'll sign up for a month's membership with a local gym, just so I can utilize different equipment and experience greater diversity in my exercise routines.

AEROBICS

I break a sweat with a stationary gym bike. I use an elliptical machine in my gym and prefer to do my running on a treadmill, since it absorbs the shock of running much better than asphalt, which can be brutal on the legs, feet and joints. If you do buy home gym equipment, it's worth saving up for sturdier equipment that can take a pounding. The cheap stuff is a poor investment in the long run. Get some opinions and feedback from friends, or the most knowledgeable person you can find at your local gym.

Another useful workout tool is a rebounder. A rebounder is a mini-trampoline that lets you work up a sweat safely, and it can be fun, too. Your workout can be as low-impact as you like. If you fatigue easily, this might be a good option for you.

For real fun, I like to work out on my heavy punching bag. I use lightweight boxing gloves or my fingerless weight lifting gloves. There's nothing like the satisfaction of hammering that bag. I can imagine it's anyone I want it to be. To heighten the fantasy, I listen to a custom CD I made with a music soundtrack, crowd noises and an announcer. The background music, a driving base-beat that's perfect for boxing, is set to loop every two minutes so I can do two-minute rounds. One tip: do not hang your heavy bag directly beneath your wife's upstairs china hutch. The reverberations from hammering the bag can ripple throughout the house's substructure and rattle the dishes and nerves of everyone inside.

EXERCISE FOR THE BODY AND THE MIND

I've got a yoga mat and a DVD on tai chi—one of these days I may actually use them. Meditative exercises are really very good ways to work out by strengthening the mind and body in parallel. Years ago, I was a fairly accomplished practitioner of yoga and taking up yoga again is part of my master plan.

COMPUTERS

You can't exactly surf the internet or build electronic spreadsheets without a computer, but you still can lose weight and reclaim your health without one. If you do have a computer, use it to become a better, stronger, and healthier person, not as something to sit in front of all day long.

Oh yes, there's one other computer I need to mention. I'm talking about the one between your ears: your brain. That lump of grey matter that fills up what would otherwise be an empty space for rent, is without a doubt the most important tool in your arsenal. Like your muscles, it too can go flabby and limp, so you've got to keep it toned. Repeat after me: "Read, think and learn; read, think and learn." Do that often enough and your brain will be as taut and brawny as the rest of your body.

Exercise does a body good, but only if that body is properly fueled. After years of eating all the foods that were wrong for me, I had to learn through trial and error, what worked best. One of the most important things I learned is that food is so much more than just fuel for the body. The food we eat is part of our cultural identity, a link to our past and a path to our future. The quality of our food plays a significant role in the quality of our lives. Is it any wonder, then, that at one time in our collective history food was sacred?

Part Four
It's All About The Food

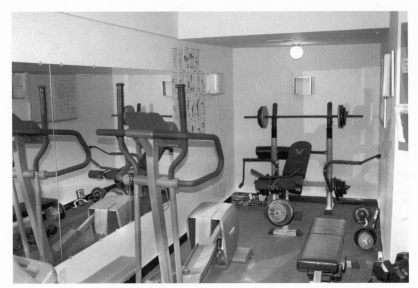

A home gym can be set up in any size room. The goal is to create a space that is dedicated to exercise--just as a kitchen is dedicated to cooking or a home theatre is dedicated to entertainment.

Chapter Eleven

When Food Was Sacred

Remembering when food was once an
important part of our lives

In 1979 while I was in college, I borrowed $300.00 and bought my first car, a pea green, four-door 1970 Datsun. The previous owners accessorized the sickly paint job with a collection of dents that covered the car like chicken pox. The rear end had been smashed in an accident, making the trunk nearly unusable. The tires were bald, the stick shift flopped about dangerously and sometimes popped out of gear of its own accord, engine fumes leaked into the passenger compartment, and occasionally the car suffered a seizure and shook so violently that it was impossible to steer.

Like most college students, I was a pauper and could not afford many of life's little extras. I had to save money wherever I could and one of the ways I saved was on gas. I generally gassed up at stations where you were likely to find more gas in a stewpot of beans than in the station pumps. I'm not saying the proprietors of these fine establishments watered down their gas, but judging by all the knocking, stalling and backfiring that ensued, I came to the conclusion that my gas tank contained more than just fossil fuels.

To make ends meet, I worked a part-time job at a large print shop. One day, at the end of my shift, my car ran out of gas in the parking lot. One of the forklift drivers came over and offered to give me enough gas to get home. He disappeared around a corner and came back a few moments later with a large fuel can. This was the same gas we used in the company trucks and it was the good stuff, premium quality, the fuel equivalent of a fine wine.

The car started up immediately. That didn't happen very often. On my way home, I noticed the car ran smoother than it had ever run before. The engine fairly purred. As I sat at a stoplight and marveled at the low throaty growl of what sounded like a high performance engine, I closed my eyes and imagined I was driving a Mercedes or some other luxury dream machine. My ancient, ailing Datsun, a true automotive embarrassment, was now transformed into a prowling cat of a car, quick off the line and tight in the turns. As there was only enough fuel to get me to a gas station near my home, those dreams vanished quickly. Once I topped off the tank with the cheap anemic gas that I normally purchased, the ghost of my old car returned with the familiar knocking, back firing, and always inconvenient stalls.

Now consider the human body. We need food the way our cars need fuel. When we put poor quality fuel in our cars, we see that decision reflected in poor performance, breakdowns and costly repair bills. The same is true of our bodies. Poor-quality food yields similarly poor physical and mental performance. The difference is that in us this inferior performance, manifests as aches and pains, lethargy, mental fog, obesity and a variety of illnesses. Anyone who cares about their car won't try to find the lowest quality fuel to put into it. They understand that doing so, over time, can have a ruinous effect on the life of the engine. The same is true for us.

If you want to increase your personal mileage in life and take on the tight turns the world sometimes throws at you, if you want to barrel down the straightway, and when your time comes to cross the finish line, if you want to look back on your life and say with conviction that yours was a race well run, you had better start filling up on the right fuel now.

Chapter Eleven: When Food Was Sacred

. . . .

FOOD AS SOCIAL RITUAL

When I was growing up, the nurturing, preparation and consumption of food was once an important part of our lives. In our home, the value of self-reliance meant that it was just as essential for the boys to know how to cook as the girls. Our Thanksgiving meals were elaborate affairs requiring days of preparation. Even on regular days, food was rarely taken lightly. Food was sacred then, and the preparation of a meal was considered tangible evidence of love for one's fellow man. The food we ate was woven into the fabric of our social behavior. It gave meaning to the notable events of our lives and was a cornerstone of our cultural heritage.

When illness struck, our mothers were more likely to head for the kitchen than to the doctor or pharmacy. Reliance on aspirin and bottled cold remedies was rare in those days. The front line of our defense against ill health came in the form of citrus teas of boiled grapefruit and black pepper, chicken soup or—the nuclear weapon of home healing—jellied bone broth, simmered for hours over a slow flame. Our mothers were live-in medical residents and their medicine cabinet was the kitchen cupboard. A teaspoon of cod liver oil was a regular, and unpleasant, accompaniment to our daily routine.

When I was about five years old, I came down with the mumps, an illness characterized by painful swelling of the salivary glands toward the back of each cheek. My mother prepared a heated poultice which was wrapped beneath my chin and knotted atop my head. The unmistakable smell of sardines gave me a clue about what it contained, but to this day, I do not know all the ingredients. The important point is that with this remedy and a diet of revitalizing soup, I was soon my old self again. This was in 1965, two years before the mumps vaccine was licensed and widely administered.

When Mary was a child, she and a number of her siblings came down with whooping cough. They were promptly quarantined from the rest of the family and put on a rigorous regimen of soup. Their throats were so sore, there was little else they could eat. As their health returned, their strength was further boosted with a delicious diet of fat and protein in the form of scrambled eggs.

Although the whole country was in a state of transition where food was concerned, our family still maintained a sense of harmony with the natural world. We ate produce in season and harbored little expectation for ripe tomatoes in the dead of winter. The Southwest had a long growing season, but we still had to wait until the oranges and sweet pink grapefruits were in season. The culture of convenience and instant gratification had not fully taken over. We accepted a slower pace of life where food was concerned, even if we did not understand its importance.

The milestones in our lives had their own special traditions and their own foods. In our community, elaborate wedding receptions were rare. After the cake had been cut, the bouquet tossed, and the happy couple had motored off to parts unknown, the wedding was over. Funerals were another matter altogether. After a funeral, it was customary to bring a dish, something cooked in your own kitchen, and gather at the home of the bereaved. There, the tears of the morning's sorrowful events were replaced by warm embraces and sincere expressions of sympathy in one corner of the house and boisterous laughter in another. Food was at the center of these events. People usually brought their favorite dishes and though the food was ostensibly intended for the bereaved, there was always more than enough to feed a houseful of sympathetic family and friends. Food after a funeral was a salve, a tangible sign that warmth and comfort could still be found in a world gone cold with the loss of a loved one.

It would have been unthinkable to bring a bucket of heat-n-eat frozen chicken to a funeral reception. In our home, the same was true for birthday cakes. Our cakes were baked from scratch. I was overcome with a sense of anticipation when I watched my mother bake a cake. There was the flour, the eggs, and the folding of the batter, followed by that painful period as we waited for the layers to bake. There was always the inevitable jockeying to see who got first dibs on licking the sweet batter from the beaters. The entire house was filled with the sweet scent of freshly baked cake. First one, then two, and finally three flat disks of sweet bread were stacked three and often four layers high on a plate. Sometimes, the layers came out of the oven uneven, but my mother, an accomplished pastry engineer, knew how to shore up an uneven cake with strategically placed toothpicks that became the focus of seek-and-find games when it was time to cut the cake.

The best part of baking a cake was the decoration. Real butter and sugar with chocolate or coconut were mixed together to create a blissfully delicious icing. If I hadn't nagged my mother too incessantly, I got to help ice the cake and even finish off the remnants in the bowl. To the layer of icing she would add decorative walnuts, or chopped coconut. These cakes were culinary masterpieces compared to the manufactured, oversized slabs of store-bought cakes available today. Decorated with partially hydrogenated vegetable oil mixed with sugar, and suspect dyes, they may be appealing to the eye, but these cakes are devoid of character, of any sense of the unique. More important than the taste was what my mother's cakes represented. Those homemade birthday cakes were a tangible expression of her love for me. The store-bought slabs that pass for cake today are a symbol of too many modern parent-child relationships—superficial style and little substance.

Many children today have never seen their mothers bake a cake or their parents actually cook real food for them. They come home to packaged noodles they prepare themselves in the microwave or eat dry out of the bag. That personal connection with a parent made possible through food does not exist in their lives. This makes for a sad commentary on the state of relationships; for what does it mean when one person says to another, in deeds if not in words, "You are not important enough for me to cook you a meal?" When the sustenance of our bodies is left to strangers, where then can we look when seeking to sustain our hearts and our minds?

A Life Unburdened

. . . .

EVERYDAY FOOD, EVERYDAY PEOPLE

Not that many years ago, food played an important part in our social traditions. From the youngest children to the weathered grandmothers, the cultural role of food in our lives was as vital to our existence as our faith. The following is a short list of how food was intertwined with the social customs of my youth.

- Young children playing house would often pretend to cook food as they understood at an early age that cooking and eating home-prepared foods was a component of the glue that holds families together.
- Preparing a dish, or perhaps dinner, for the first time was a rite of passage.
- While a young man asking a young lady out to dinner was clear evidence of a romantic interest, if she cooked for him, that was an order of magnitude more serious.
- Birthday cakes were baked from scratch because no one could bake as well as mom.
- Homemade, hand-cranked ice cream was a rare treat that was always regarded as superior to store-bought ice cream.
- It was considered a sin to waste food.
- Home-cooked meals were considered superior to all others.
- Women and men bragged about their cooking skills.
- Cooking was considered a necessary skill.

We may have lacked many things in those days, but we ate good food, and, like my old Datsun running on good gas, we were healthier for it. Without a full-time working automobile, money for cabs or even buses, we walked most places. But the food we ate was satisfying and provided the nutrients needed to fuel a day's worth of tasks. Overweight people were rare in those days. We saw obese people at the "freak shows" staged just off the main midway at the county fair. There, for the price of a bag of popcorn, one could gawk at the fat lady or the fat man, and marvel at the expansive capacity of the human body. Now all one need do is go to the mall or look in the mirror. This is progress?

Food used to be simple, but not anymore. The burden of trying to decide what we should eat has turned meal planning into a science project. A quick look at a typical list of ingredients helps explain why. Over the course of two years, I had to relearn a few of the simple things about food, and what happens to us when we eat.

Chapter Twelve

Just the Facts About Food

A few simple things about food that made
all the difference for my family

There is actually nothing simple about food anymore. The typical grocery store has thousands of items for sale. Most of this food comes packaged in pretty containers festooned with appealing images and text. These foods often contain a worrisome list of preservatives and additives designed to make the food appear fresh. Some of the chief ingredients include sugar, grain, soy, vegetable oils and monosodium glutamate. Let's take a look at some typical foods and ingredients more closely.

SUGAR

It has been said that money makes the world go round, but I'm convinced it's sugar that keeps us spinning through the cosmos.
Sugar, and sugar substitutes, are the drug-of-choice today for both children and adults. When I was young, we had desserts made with sugar as a special treat. Not many generations before that, refined sugar was unknown.

Few who experience the taste of sugar for the first time can resist it—and that is the problem. Even in moderate amounts, sugar in all its forms can wreak holy havoc on the human system. When we think of sugar, we often think of plain old white table sugar, but practically speaking, we get sugar in a variety of forms. There's cane sugar, crystalline fructose, high fructose corn syrup (HFCS), corn syrup, honey, tree sap (maple syrup), the natural sugars found in fruits and vegetables, and lactose, the naturally occurring sugar found in milk. White flour and white rice are also a source of readily available sugar in the form of glucose.

When you eat sugar it is quickly broken down and absorbed, arriving in your bloodstream as glucose and then to be transported to your muscles for energy. If you happen to be exercising, this energy is used, but if you're sitting on the couch giving your thumb a workout on the TV remote, any glucose that exceeds the carrying capacity of the liver and muscles is stored in your adipose tissue—this means you get fatter. This whole process requires many vitamins and minerals, but refined sugar provides none of these, so the body has to use nutrients that it has stored. Eating refined sugars is like going to the bank everyday to withdraw money without ever making a deposit. Soon your body—like your bank account—becomes depleted.

Another problem with refined sugars is that they are metabolized very quickly, shooting straight to your bloodstream. Your blood sugar goes up, triggering an energy burst and even a drug-like "high." This blood glucose spike triggers an insulin response—insulin gets sugar out of the bloodstream by moving it into the cells—as your body brings the level of glucose back to normal. Then, as blood glucose levels drop, you get the inevitable "low" in the form of lethargy and a lack of energy. That's when you feel hungry and the cravings begin. You wind up overeating because a diet unbalanced toward simple sugars leaves you hungry more often. If you're not running marathons, all of this excess glucose ultimately gets converted to stored energy as fat. The result is that you gain lots and lots of weight.

If this process goes on too long, your body can become less sensitive to insulin, a condition called insulin resistance. If your body continues under siege in this manner, you risk developing Type 2 diabetes, a condition in which the body becomes very insensitive to insulin. This means that your blood will be awash in sugar, but your cells will be starving. . . no wonder so many people don't feel like exercising!

Chapter Twelve: Just the Facts About Food

Under these conditions, even sources of sugar normally regarded as healthy—like whole grains and fruits—may supply more glucose than the body can efficiently handle. Type 2 diabetics tend to gain lots of weight, especially around the middle. They may even develop Type 1 diabetes. Type 1 diabetics lose the ability to produce insulin altogether. When this happens, rapid weight loss typically follows, because without insulin, the body becomes very inefficient at storing fat. Type 1 diabetics must rely on insulin injections to make up for the insulin their bodies can no longer produce.

THE BODY FACTORY

Simple sugars provide energy but very little nutritive value. If you think of your digestive system as a factory and the various components as machines, there are associated costs with running those machines. In a real factory, those costs would constitute the operating overhead that includes electricity, personnel, machine maintenance, etc. Your digestive machinery, as well as all of your interdependent biological systems, has an operating overhead as well. Everything from the production of saliva, enzymes and stomach acid to the digestive musculature that moves food along the system exerts a cost in terms of energy and the expenditure of nutrients.

A manager of a real factory would never go in every Sunday and turn on the lights and all the machines when there were no products being produced. Without products, there can be no sales and no revenue. The costs of running the factory without producing any products would eat into the company's overall profits and could eventually bankrupt the company. Likewise, a diet high in simple sugars that provides few nutrients is an expensive proposition that provides little return on the investment of running your body's interdependent systems. Ultimately, you may find yourself filing for bankruptcy in the form of obesity, diabetes and heart disease.

GOING AGAINST THE GRAIN

Refined grains used in donuts, pastries and bread behave much the same as sugar. This means eating a slice of white bread is metabolically equivalent to eating sugar. White flour is what is left over after whole grains have been stripped of their vitamins, minerals and fiber. Without these nutrients, refined grains are more easily and quickly digested. The net effect is the same as eating sugar, namely a quick rush of sugar into the bloodstream. I discovered that my cravings for sweet foods remained high as long as my consumption of refined grains remained high. When I scaled back on both sugar and grains, I saw the cravings subside. I have since all but eliminated added sugars from my diet. The sugar I do consume comes in the form of fructose, found in fruits and some vegetables, lactose, found in dairy products, and the rare treat sweetened with raw honey or maple syrup, two sweeteners that still have all their vitamins and minerals.

What about whole grains? I eat very little grain, but when I do, it's whole grain. However, I discovered that while whole grains are clearly better for me than refined grains, they still exerted a dampening effect on my physical and emotional well being. Over-consumption leaves me feeling lethargic, so I don't eat even whole grains that much. After nearly two years of eating small amounts of whole grain foods, I find that I no longer crave sugar or grains.

SOY

I was once an ardent admirer and consumer of soy foods. I believed in the much-hyped message about the healthful benefits of soy. I ate tofu straight out of the package, in all its flavorless splendor. I consumed soy protein shakes, soy meat and a host of other synthetic foods made from this "miraculous" substance, credited with curing everything from cancer to baldness.

Soy is a potent source of isoflavones, compounds that mimic the effects of estrogen, a female hormone. While the industry claims that these isoflavones are beneficial, they have actually been linked to thyroid problems. . . and a consequence of low thyroid function is weight gain and persistent fatigue. Even worse, a university study showed that men who were subjected to mega-doses of soy experienced breast enlargement, nipple discharge and a reduction in testosterone production. Yet the newspapers touted this study as proof that men should eat more soy!

Soy has been marketed as a miracle health food for years, but this has more to do with the fact that the soy industry spends millions promoting soy products than the fact that soy has any inherent health value. A cursory look at the research reveals a troubling list of health problems from soy. I recommend *The Whole Soy Story: The Dark Side of America's Favorite Health Food*, by Kaayla Daniel, a book that will open your eyes to the downside of soy.

In Asia, soy used for anything other than a flavoring was considered a cheap poverty food; in the U.S., it has been used as a cheap animal food. But the industry has cleverly marketed cheap imitation foods based on soy as high-end health foods. There's irony here in that really high end foods and ingredients—like saffron, truffles, fois gras and expensive wines—are quite rare on the average American's table.

One of the claims made for soy is that it is "natural." This is true only insofar as everything on planet earth derived from raw materials is natural. What is unnatural are the frightening synthetic foods soy is used to create. Soy "milk," soy "meat," soy "cheese"—the list of fake foods grows every day. What's worse is that these faux foods come bundled with troubling amounts of sugar, MSG, refined grains, additives and preservatives.

Never in the history of the human race have people consumed as much soy as we do today. Half the space in the dairy case in many grocery stores is taken up by soy products. Babies are given soy milk. School lunch programs now include foods "enhanced" with soy, and most processed foods contain soy as an ingredient. What is frightening is that no one knows what effect a dietary change of this magnitude will have on the populace over time. In animals, being fed lots of soy leads to fertility problems. While traditional fermented soy foods—the kind of foods Asian societies have been consuming for centuries—are historically safe when consumed in small amounts, over-consumption of processed soy foods may represent a Pandora's box of unpleasant surprises 20 or 30 years from now. . . or even sooner

Despite my devotion to soy, I found it to be incompatible with a healthy diet. When I exorcised soy from my diet and converted to real food, many of the dietary demons that had haunted me for more than a decade were vanquished.

FATS AND OILS

I do not avoid fat, but I'm careful to eat only the right kind. That means mostly animal fats, the traditional fats that have sustained humans for thousands of years—real butter, lard rendered from healthy, humanely raised pigs, whole dairy products, whole eggs from pastured chickens, the fat on my meat and good old fashioned cod liver oil. As for the oils that come from plants, I use coconut oil and a little olive oil. Nutrition professionals will tell you that you shouldn't consume these fats because, with the exception of olive oil, they're bad for your heart. This position defies logic because for thousands of years human consumption of these fats was commonplace and heart disease was practically unknown. What was really bad for my heart was carrying around an extra 200 pounds that I couldn't get rid of because of a low-fat, processed food diet that left me undernourished, enervated and depressed.

When I was younger, my mother used to render lard by boiling fatback. When she was in her 40s, her doctor told her she would die of heart failure in a year or two, yet she lived a vigorous and full life well into her 70s. She died several days after paying a long delayed visit to a doctor where she was subjected to a round of supposedly "necessary" inoculations.

Chapter Twelve: Just the Facts About Food

. . . .

For an eye-opening, science-based explanation of why the cholesterol and saturated fat theory of disease doesn't hold up, read *The Cholesterol Myths*, by Dr. Uffe Ravnskov.

A few decades ago, we were advised to switch from healthy animal fats to vegetable oils. We were told that these mostly polyunsaturated oils were healthier for us. Yet highly polyunsaturated vegetable oils are full of what's called free radicals, the real culprit in cancer and heart disease. When these liquid oils go through a process to make them hardened—called partial hydrogenation—trans fats are formed. Like the free radicals in vegetable oils, trans fats contribute to cancer, heart disease and many other ailments.

There are many good scientific reasons for eating traditional fats. Animal fats provide important nutrients you can't get anywhere else, including one called CLA (conjugated linoleic acid) in the fat of grass-fed animals. CLA has been shown to help the body lose fat and build muscle. Lard is a great source of vitamin D. As for coconut oil, the body uses this extraordinary fat for quick energy and never stores it in the fatty tissues. Coconut oil also boosts thyroid function, making it a great fat for weight loss. The good fats in coconut oil are all saturated fats. When the anti-saturated fat hysteria came along, the food industry was forced to switch from using lard and coconut oil to partially hydrogenated vegetable oils loaded with trans fats.

I love to cook with coconut oil because it provides an excellent source of energy, adds tons of flavor to food and acts as an appetite suppressant, which helps to spur weight loss.

If you want to know more about coconut oil and its healthy role in diet and weight loss, read *Eat Fat, Lose Fat*, by Dr. Mary G. Enig and Sally Fallon. Another book, *Know Your Fats: The Complete Primer for Understanding the Nutrition of Fats, Oils and Cholesterol*, by Dr. Enig, is the most comprehensive, unbiased and accurate book on the science of dietary fat available to the public.

As for olive oil, I consume small amounts of extra virgin olive oil that is packaged in dark bottles (to protect the oil from light) and minimally processed. I keep olive oil in a dark cool spot in the pantry, and buy small bottles so that it doesn't sit around for too long. I never cook with olive oil, instead using it as a flavor enhancer on salads and for making homemade mayonnaise.

MONOSODIUM GLUTAMATE

Monosodium glutamate, or MSG, is a manufactured free glutamic acid that is used to enhance the flavor of some of your favorite foods. While the FDA allows the use of MSG in many foods, ongoing research suggests that MSG may react negatively with the human nervous system. The FDA has accordingly identified MSG as a chemical worthy of further study. Animal studies have shown that MSG can cause brain damage yet it still shows up in baby foods disguised as hydrolyzed protein. Some of the symptoms experienced by people sensitive to MSG include headaches, chest pain, nausea, drowsiness and weakness. Most interesting is the fact that MSG given to growing animals makes them obese! You don't need a degree in food science, chemistry or endocrinology to realize that MSG is an additive that should be avoided.

A significant problem with manufactured free glutamates is that their presence in food is not always easy to discern, as they may be listed under a number of euphemistic aliases including hydrolyzed protein, autolyzed yeast extract, flavors, natural flavors, broth and sodium caseinate. The elimination of processed foods from your diet will eliminate manufactured free glutamates from your life.

ARTIFICIAL SWEETENERS

Industry's acknowledgement of the hazards of excess sugar in the diet is reflected in the growing number of artificial sweeteners on the market. However, concern for dietary sugar has mostly been limited to the calories it contains and its effect on weight. Saccharine (Sweet 'N Low), sucralose (Splenda), aspartame (NutraSweet and Equal) and a number of other contenders have vied for the top spot as America's replacement for sugar. Disagreement about the health and safety of artificial sweeteners has kept pace with their development.

An important point about artificial sweeteners—a point often overlooked—is the amount of sweets necessary for a satisfying diet. The assumption seems to be that we need a lot of sweets in our diet. The sensory appeal of sugar and its substitutes is undeniable, but I believe that appeal has been exaggerated out of proportion by diets overloaded with sweet tasting foods. I discovered that replacing sugar with sugar substitutes did little to curb my cravings for sweet foods. In some cases, because the substitutes never tasted as good as regular sugar, my cravings for the real thing were even stronger. I realized that my threshold for detecting sweetness was distorted and that by consuming sugar substitutes, I was maintaining an abnormally high level of desire for sweet foods.

Research suggests that sugar substitutes interfere with the body's ability to regulate caloric intake, leading to greater consumption and weight gain. Once I cut out artificial sweeteners altogether and replaced them with small amounts of natural sugar from raw honey and maple syrup, my "satisfaction-threshold" for sweetness dropped dramatically! Sugary drinks became too sweet for my taste and when I do consume something sweet—like fruit or ice cream sweetened with honey—a little bit goes a long, long way.

WHY ARE WE SICK?

It should be apparent by now that many of us are eating large quantities of foods that our bodies are not designed to accommodate. Critics of this view protest that all foods are equal, and suggest that our digestive systems are little more than hollow, biological garbage disposals through which we can flush all manner of junk food without fear of any ill effect, save weight gain.

They claim that those who warn about the dangers of an unhealthy diet are scaremongers, and that exercise is a panacea for all our problems. Actually, the true scaremongers are those who would seek to deprive us of our right to accurate information on nutrition and the ability to choose what we eat. They do this by undermining the political process through industry-funded "influence" on our elected officials and government agencies.

Is food the cause of many of our health problems today? Food is not the sole cause, but it is certainly a major contributor. What could have more impact on our health than what we put into our bodies every single day? To suggest otherwise is to separate oneself from reason and good common sense.

Chapter Thirteen

What I Eat
A look inside my pantry at the foods that changed my life

I eat whole, pastured meats, including beef, chicken, pork, fish and turkey. I get much of my meat from local farmers who properly care for their animals. I've found that grass-fed, pastured beef is far better for me than grain-fed. The chicken and turkey are pastured as well, and the pork comes from a trusted source.

I believe the quality of the meat I eat is very important, and you should, too. Check your local area for suppliers of high-quality meat. When the grocery store is my only option, I buy regular meat, but I do not buy processed meats like sliced turkey, ham and beef. These meats are often loaded with MSG and sometimes sugar. When I do buy meat from a grocery store, I shop in the section where the butcher resides. If you have the resources consider purchasing a half or one quarter of pastured beef. You'll need plenty of storage, but the price break you receive for buying in bulk makes it worthwhile to pick up an extra freezer.

Once when I was child our home was burglarized. We found that the usual items had been taken: a camera, radio and a few other small electronics. What surprised us was the discovery that several packages of steak, from a side of packaged beef we kept in the freezer, were missing. It seems that even petty thieves understand the importance of nutrient-dense foods.

I also enjoy organ meats, principally liver, and eat it several times a month. Cow's liver is nutrient dense, and cooked properly, that is to say rare, it is delicious. I buy wild-caught salmon when I can get it, but will settle for farmed in a pinch. I have found sardines to be an excellent seafood source, and take tins with me when I travel.

RAW DAIRY

Imprison a milk cow in a confined space, force her to stand on concrete, keep her strung out on hormones and antibiotics, and feed her nothing but grain, soy, and bakery refuse. How can you expect her milk to be nourishing? I've touched on this point before, but I want to talk about one of the foods that has been essential in my recovery. Milk from these "factory" cows is then pasteurized and homogenized to produce a beverage that is nutritionally inferior, difficult to digest and uniformly bland throughout the year. This triumph of "consistent mediocrity" is regarded as a success by the industrial milk industry.

Pasteurized milk is milk that has been quickly brought to high heat to kill off dangerous pathogens that may be lurking in the milk. This is a necessary step with commercial milk from factory farmed cows, which is typically brimming with pathogens. Unfortunately, pasteurization also kills off the beneficial bacteria and enzymes in the milk, making all the nutrients more difficult to absorb and turning it into little more than dead, white water. Actually, most milk today, including "organic" milk, is ultra-pasteurized, that is, brought to a temperature above the boiling point in just a few seconds. More and more people simply can't tolerate commercial milk. I can't. It literally makes me sick.

The alternative is milk from a family farm cow lucky enough to live on green pasture. In fact, the healthiest milk (and butter, cream and cheese) comes from cows eating new grass, growing at an accelerated rate in the spring and early fall. Taken in raw form, milk from these cows is full-bodied, much creamier, easy to digest and incredibly delicious. The fast-growing grass is more nutrient-dense and undoubtedly more delicious to the cows. Butter made from this milk is flavorful and has a rich golden color and an aroma you can smell from across the room. By comparison, conventional butter from pasteurized milk has no aroma at all. But the real difference is in the nutrients. Butter from cows eating grass has much, much more.

Whipped cream, cheese and ice cream made with milk from cows eating green grass is unparalleled in flavor and texture. Once you partake of this ambrosia, you come to understand the origin of the phrase "living off the fat of the land."

My personal preference is for raw milk products, including un-pasteurized, unhomogenized milk. I consume cheese, butter, cream and yogurt made from raw milk as well. Raw milk—Nature's perfect food—may not be an option for everyone as liquid raw milk products are hard to come by due to pressure from the dairy industry.

Raw milk is actually quite safe, as long as the farmer follows reasonable standards of cleanliness, because raw milk contains many components that kill off harmful bacteria. In addition, raw milk directly purchased from a pasture-based farm comes from cows allowed to graze on grass, not kept confined in sheds and given growth hormones. Because these cows eat the food they were designed to eat—grass—they are typically disease-free, reducing or eliminating the need for antibiotics.

Finding a source may be difficult, but it is well worth the effort to look for one. The web site realmilk.com lists local sources in your area including milk available through cow-share and herd-share arrangements. A cow-share program allows you to become a co-owner of a cow. This gives you the right to drink the milk from your cow in states that prohibit the sale of raw milk. You can even order raw milk from farmers who will ship it to you frozen.

It is a sad commentary on the state of the nation when citizens who choose to purchase good, clean, healthful and delicious raw milk are prohibited from doing so by an overzealous regulatory system that fears the healthy competition that raw milk sales represent. Raw milk may not be for everyone, but everyone should have the right to drink it if they choose.

EGGS, WONDERFUL EGGS

Like many people, I was deathly afraid of eggs. I believed the myth that they were dangerous due to their supposedly unhealthy combination of dietary fat and cholesterol. I still liked eggs, and so resorted to some of the egg substitutes available at the time. I found that if it looks like an egg, and cooks like an egg, it won't necessarily taste like an egg. To put it mildly, I was underwhelmed by the egg substitutes I tried. I later learned that when egg substitutes are fed as the only food to rats, they die very quickly.

In time I discovered that blood cholesterol levels are minimally affected by dietary cholesterol, and that the theory of cholesterol as a primary cause of heart disease is unsupported when you examine the science. Now I eat eggs often. They really are a perfect food. My preference is for pastured eggs, which are eggs from chickens that spend lots of time on grass, socializing, exercising, developing a pecking order and eating greens and bugs. I've found that the darker the egg yolk, the more flavorful and nutritious the egg. Spring yolks from pastured chickens are deliciously dark—almost orange. Conventional egg yolks are woefully pale in color and taste, by comparison. Nevertheless, I much prefer conventional eggs to egg substitutes, which I can no longer abide.

I am somewhat skeptical of terms like "free range" and "cage free," as I've found these eggs to be only marginally better than conventional ones, as far as taste and color are concerned. I have learned that these eggs come from hens that "roam" in large barns—not in cages, but not outdoors either. If you're going to pay premium prices for any eggs, the first choice should be pastured eggs directly from a farmer. My second choice would be "free range," "cage free," or omega 3 enhanced. How you eat your eggs is up to you. Whether you like them poached, fried in butter or bacon fat, scrambled in omelets or hard boiled, it's all good eating.

SOUPS AND BROTH

Two of our favorite foods to eat when the weather turns chilly are soups and broths. A hearty chicken or beef soup that has been allowed to slow-cook all day fills the house with a wonderful aroma as it soothes the body and the soul. We allow broths to simmer for up to 24 hours or more. Once chilled, the broth changes from a liquid to a gelatin-like consistency. It has been our experience that broth made from the typical big-box grocery store chicken will not gel sufficiently, suggesting a thinness of character to match the deficit of nutrients from these factory farmed "jailbirds." Do not be dissuaded, however, from making your own broth from the chickens you normally buy, as home made broth always trumps the store bought variety, which often comes loaded with MSG. Broth serves a number of uses. It is loaded with nutrients, is delicious and from our own experience, possesses curative properties. It can be heated and eaten as is or added to a variety of dishes to enhance their flavor.

FRESH PRODUCE

Anyone who has ever purchased produce has encountered the attractive piece of fruit that fails the taste test. When I was a child, it was customary for my family to purchase a large box of red delicious apples during the holiday season. We put these apples out on the back porch where the chill evening air kept them crisp and fresh tasting. It was unusual to find a bad apple in those days. Sadly, the opposite is true today, where finding a red delicious apple that lives up to the second half of its name is a challenge.

Fresh vegetables and fruit are a must in any healthy diet. I eat far more vegetables than fruit, as I've found that less is best when it comes to sweet foods. Finding good quality organic produce is easy, as it is available in many stores these days. Organically labeled produce is nice to have, but don't pass up locally grown produce which, even if it isn't labeled as organic, may be just as good, if not better. Even regular conventionally grown fruits and vegetables are superior to anything in the snack food aisle, so don't let the lack of an organic label deter you.

One of the problems with produce in general, and conventional produce in particular, is that growers tend to emphasize size and color over taste. The nutritional profile of conventional produce is usually a low priority. The nutrients found in produce are derived from the soil in which they grow. Nutrient poor soil equals nutrient poor produce. Poor soil management practices favored by some growers have resulted in produce with suboptimal nutritional profiles. This diminished quality in the food we eat is the price we pay for getting what we want exactly when we want it, in or out of season.

Buying produce when it's in season is the best time to buy because the prices will be lower and the quality higher. Community Supported Agriculture programs (CSAs) and farmers' markets are an economical alternative for this very reason. While you can save money on conventional produce from the grocery store when items are on sale, your savings are limited by the fact that some of that produce may not be of the best quality.

Local farmers' markets are good places to buy produce, but don't assume that just because the guy operating the produce stand is wearing jeans and a straw hat that you're getting high quality locally grown produce. If it's November in North Dakota and you find bananas and strawberries at the farmers' market, you can be sure those fruits were not locally grown. When in doubt, be sure to ask. Buying imported produce isn't inherently bad, but fruits and vegetables grown locally and bought in season usually taste better and are more nutritious. One clue to nutritional quality is how long a piece of fruit lasts. Fruit grown in poor soil rots very quickly.

Why limit ourselves to eating in-season? After all, many nutrition experts tell us not to deprive ourselves. They say that a culture of instant gratification where nothing is off-limits is a good thing. We're told that human progress is measured not by the realization of our symbiotic relationship with the rest of life on this planet, but by whether we can get pesticide-soaked genetically modified strawberries in the dead of winter to put on our low-fat soy cheesecake.

Eating in-season helps us to relearn the virtue of patience and the value of respect for the seasonal growing cycle. Eating in season puts our bodies back in synch with the natural world from which we came. And since there's no such thing as a junk food season, eating in season teaches us to recognize what is and isn't food. In a more practical vein, produce consumed in season typically costs less than higher priced off-season produce. In addition, by buying locally, you're supporting the local economy and local growers. Of course, you can always grow your own, and it doesn't matter whether you have 40 acres or a few square feet on the back patio of a townhouse, you can grow food almost anywhere.

If you're new to growing your own, farmers' markets are a good place for the beginner to get a jump start on the season by purchasing starter plants in search of a permanent home. Simply transplant them into your garden. Generally speaking, I've found starter plants from the farmers' market to be healthier and more reliable than those found at the garden centers of large big-box stores and more successful than starting from seeds. Of course you will expend more physical effort tending your garden, but that's a good thing as the exercise will get you into the fresh air and help you lose weight. The exercise and the satisfaction of knowing that you're eating home grown, fresh, better-than-organic produce, makes that effort worthwhile.

Our garden is a raised bed contained within two rectangular boxes. Raised beds are great for small gardens because the deep soil provides plenty of extra growing space for the plant roots. Longer stronger roots yield bigger, healthier plants. We've had two seasons with our garden where we grow tomatoes, cabbage, peppers, zucchini, onions and collard greens.

LIVE FOOD/DEAD FOOD

I also eat lacto-fermented foods, like old-fashioned sauerkraut, kimchee, pickles, beet kvas (a fermented drink made from sugar beets) and kefir, which is a fermented milk beverage. Fermented foods are foods prepared traditionally with a fermenting agent like whey, which transforms the sugars into beneficial lactic acid and creates increased levels of natural enzymes and beneficial bacteria. These enzymes aid in the digestion of food. Since I've been using fermented foods, I find that I no longer get indigestion or suffer from acid reflux.

One of my favorite fermented beverages is homemade ginger ale. The first time you drink it, you realize it's not your father's ginger ale— it's your grandfather's. I make it with peeled and chopped ginger, raw honey, lime juice, and whey. It takes several days to brew and is delicious—sparkling, thirst quenching and non-alcoholic. Another favorite treat is crispy nuts. I usually use almonds or pecans and soak them overnight in salt water. After soaking, I dry them out in a food dehydrator. An oven works just as well. The result is a crispy snack that is delicious and easy to eat because soaking helps to break down the enzyme inhibitors that can make them harder to digest. You'll find recipes for lacto-fermented condiments, beverages and crispy nuts in *Nourishing Traditions*, by Sally Fallon and Mary Enig, PhD.

Humans have evolved to coexist with our environment; an environment that includes a host of beneficial bacteria that aid us in a number of ways, like the efficient digestion of our food. Unfortunately, much of the food we eat today has been stripped of its life-giving properties—foods like pasteurized milk which is essentially a dead product or pasteurized pickles. Without the aid of beneficial enzymes and bacteria, our body must work harder to carry out the metabolic operations it was designed to perform. This extra effort, under less-than-ideal circumstances wears on the body, and causes premature aging, fatigue and disease.

HOME COOKING

Chapter Thirteen: What I Eat

. . . .

One of the great tragedies of modern life is that people no longer cook for themselves. Cooking your own food allows you to control what goes into it, and you can customize your meals so that they are healthy and taste the way you want. The biggest lie the food industry has fed to the American public is the lie that we are all too busy to cook. When I consider my wife's mother, who had twelve children, and how she managed to cook meals all those years, I couldn't understand how my wife and I had so much difficulty getting a homemade meal on the table for ourselves and our two children. Fortunately, we have changed. Since our epiphany, either my wife, my daughters, or I have cooked nearly every meal we've eaten over the last two years. It took some planning initially, but it was never a matter of time so much as it was a matter of priorities.

THE OBESITY EPIDEMIC

Has an increase in the consumption of sugar, grains, and vegetable oils led to an increase in obesity? Yes, it has. Let's look at the state of food today:

- There are vending machines in public schools, in the workplace and even in hospitals, that weren't there a few decades ago.
- Fast food eateries exist on practically every corner now, and can even be found in hospitals. In some inner city neighborhoods, the only food you can buy is fast food because there are no grocery stores.
- People used to take the time to bake their own cakes for birthdays. Now you can purchase a massive slab of cake, personalized with a special message, for relatively little money and virtually no time at all.
- The pricing structure for junk food is such that for a small increase in price, a customer receives a significantly larger increase in the amount of food.
- Government subsidies for corn and soy has fueled explosive growth in the manufacture and availability of cheap junk foods.

- Junk food advertising to adults and children has increased dramatically.
- While gas, housing and transportation costs have risen over the years, the price of processed convenience food has remained affordable or has even decreased.
- Portion sizes served in restaurants, and included in ready-to eat convenience foods have increased.
- In every bus station, train station and airport, you can find low cost junk and processed foods with ease, while something as simple as fresh fruit or real cheese is extremely difficult to find.
- Despite the fact that real food amounts to little more than produce, meat and dairy products, there are thousands of new convenience foods available that didn't even exist 50 years ago.
- Breakfast has degenerated from meat and eggs to sugared cereals to donuts to candy bars. Each succesive generation in the devolution of breakfast is higher in calories and lower in nutrients.
- Most of the foods in the grocery store have sugar, grain (corn, wheat and rice) and processed fats and oils as key ingredients.
- It is possible today to buy 50 pieces of fried chicken for little more than $25.00 at some retail outlets. Most of the calories in that chicken come from the breading and the frying oil.

It is an exercise in self-delusion to claim that the modern diet has not caused our current health crisis. The rate of obesity did not double over the last thirty years because people were eating too much fruit, vegetables, meat and whole grains. It doubled because of the reasons stated above, along with a lack of exercise.

In the first half of 2003, my diet and that of my family was as bad as it could be. We were sick and were growing more ill each day. Something had to change. They say that when you reach the end of your rope, you only have two options: let go or start climbing. We decided to climb.

Chapter Fourteen

The Total Food Index
A common sense tool to help you decide what you should eat

I've recently learned that there is a category of foods designed to be consumed unconsciously. Put simply, this class of foods is eaten without thinking, like when you're navigating rush hour traffic, simultaneously juggling a phone in one hand and a quarter-pound burger and fries in the other. Many people will consume this pre-dinner "meal" in their car without thinking, then sit down to dinner once they get home. That's the magic of these foods. You eat more because you're not fully conscious of what and when you're eating. Our homes, cars and offices are often full of snack foods that we blindly consume throughout the day. The last thing junk food companies want is for you to actually start thinking about what you eat. Tracking your food neutralizes one of their most potent weapons against you.

But isn't tracking what you eat a lot of work? Food tracking is not for everyone, but it is useful for some people. Look at this way: you can continue to be a snack zombie for the food industry or you can wrest back control of your life with this simple, powerful tool. I never would have had any success without this technique. Its power lies in the fact that it stops unconscious eating dead in its tracks. Once you start writing down what you eat before you eat, you will never again put another morsel of food into your mouth without thinking about it first. This technique is an real eye-opener. You may find that you're putting away far more calories or doing much more snacking than you realized. This brief moment of awareness can make all the difference between inhaling a bag of chips and developing the motivation and the good sense not to.

For those people who say, "but I really don't eat that much," consider this: I was socking away well over 5000 calories a day at one point but never realized it. I actually believed I was a light eater most days. The simple fact is that it's awfully hard to pack on 100 extra pounds without eating a whole lot of high-calorie food.

It is true that as your body becomes more efficient at fat storage, the less you need to eat to gain weight. Still, tracking gives you a baseline of where you're starting from and helps you to see patterns between what and when you eat, your mood and other behavioral signals that can clue you in to some of the underlying emotional, physical and situational reasons behind your eating behavior. If you're eating a good balance of nutritious whole foods, don't obsess over macronutrients. The goal is to determine what your eating patterns were like before transitioning to a whole foods plan, and how they changed afterward.

The good news is that this is not something you'll have to do for the rest of your life. For many people, it may simply be a good place to start.

WHICH FOODS SHOULD YOU EAT?

Once you get past the propaganda of "no bad foods," you have to decide which foods you should eat, which foods you should cut back on and which foods to cut out of your diet. I devised a method for determining which foods I should eat that has been very effective for me. It may be useful for you as well. I look at food as having four primary properties, which I define as the Total Food Index or TFI. The TFI rating of any food is a combination of a Nutrition Index, An accessibility Index, an Addiction Index and a Feedback Index.

The nutrition index is the first and most important factor to be considered. Your goal should be to eat the most nutritious foods, most of the time. This index works on a 10-point scale, with -5 indicating the lowest level of nutrition, and +5 the highest. The core question is, how nutritious is a particular food? Foods in the minus range are foods that represent poor nutritional choices. A food rated 'o' would be one that has a neutral or average nutritional value, like home made cookies made from whole oats and honey. They're better than commercial cookies nutritionally, but they're still not something you'd want to eat every day. On my scale, soda, which has a negative nutritional value, rates very low, with an index of −5, but raw milk, with its energizing enzymes and healthful fat, a +5. I also take into consideration the amount of preservatives and additives in a food. The more of these "extras" a food contains, the lower the nutritional score.

I rate luncheon meat, full of additives, a -2 or -3. Fresh meat gets a +2 or +3 and liver, which is a very nutrient-dense food, gets a +5. Another +5 is cod liver oil.

The accessibility index is a 10-point scale, with -5 indicating the least accessible foods and +5 being the most accessible. The core question is, how accessible is a particular food? In this case, raw milk would rate a −3, as it is not easy to find these days. Soda is everywhere, is cheap, and readily available, so it would rate a +5. Most processed convenience foods are cheap, easy to find, and easy to eat, meaning their accessibility index will usually be high. Another useful example might be a homemade dish like baked salmon. The cost of salmon, plus the fact that you have to cook it yourself, means that you're less likely to eat it everyday. Likewise, if you had baked salmon at a restaurant, the cost and the logistics involved in getting to the restaurant would mean that the accessibility index is lower. Compare the accessibility of salmon to a fried-fish sandwich at the drive-thru. Because fried fish is cheaper, precooked and conveniently located at the fast food joint down the street, the accessibility index will be higher. Ironically, many of the most nonnutritive foods tend to be the most accessible.

The addiction index is a 10-point scale with -5 indicating the least addictive foods and +5 being the most addictive. The core question is, how difficult or easy is it for me to control my consumption of this food?

If you can't be trusted around chocolate, you would give chocolate an addiction rating of +4 or +5. Beef liver from grass fed animals is a very nutritious food, but for someone who doesn't like liver, the addiction index for liver might be very low (-1 or −2) because they have no difficulty controlling their consumption. Addiction is never a good thing as it is possible to over-consume healthy foods too, so any food with a high addiction index is something you should carefully manage.

Feedback refers to how the food makes you feel emotionally, and physically. Do you get a stomachache after eating certain foods? Do some foods leave you feeling depressed, while others leave you energized? The feedback index is a 10-point scale with -5 identifying the foods with the least positive feedback and +5 indicating the most positive. I found that keeping a food journal was helpful in determining the feedback index of the foods I ate.

HOW THE TFI WORKS

The primary goal and purpose of the TFI tool is to help you learn to eat foods which are highly nutritious most of the time. It will help you cut back on foods which are moderately good for you, and eliminate those which provide poor nutrition.

Here are two examples of how I used the TFI. Nuts, like almonds, are healthy snacks. On the TFI scale for me, they rate high nutritionally (+4), and their accessibility rating is low (-3) because I have to soak them in a brine, then dry them out. The addiction index for almonds is a +2 (down from +5). I used to have great difficulty controlling consumption, so I had to cut back on preparing them. The feedback index was low initially because I found them difficult to digest. Eating them left me feeling bloated. Soaking solved that problem.

Pistachios have a high (+5) addiction index for me, so I had to cut them out completely, because I could not stop eating them and the more I ate, the more I wanted. At one time, potato chips were a high addiction food for me. I'm no longer addicted to them, but because of their low

174

nutrition rating, I don't eat them. The addiction index helps you identify these foods, regulate their consumption or get them out of your life.

One final example is homemade ice cream. I love it, but the sugar makes the nutritional index for ice cream a -1 for me. Fortunately, because it is made from real ingredients, it is a very satisfying dish, so a little goes a long, long way, which means the addiction index is very low (-4). With a low accessibility index due to the ingredients required, there's no danger of overeating. I eat about one cup a month, and I can enjoy it without worrying about my health.

Why don't I just produce a master chart that shows the TFI ratings for common foods? Wouldn't that be easier? No, because the TFI index ratings will differ from person to person. While the nutritional indexes will remain constant across the board, the accessibility, addiction, and feedback indexes may differ greatly. In addition, the TFI rating for a particular food may change over time. You may discover, as I did, that foods that were once difficult to manage are no longer a problem. The most important goal is for you to learn to make these assessments yourself. Investigate the nutritional value of the food you eat. Assess the accessibility and addictive potential of that food. Assess the feedback of the foods. How do they affect you mentally, physically, and emotionally? Learn to make the decisions that are right for you. This is the definition of nutritional empowerment.

AFTER GETTING OVER WEIGHT, WHAT'S NEXT?

Eating good food, losing weight, and exercising is great, but doing these things just for the sake of doing them seems an empty, unfulfilling exercise. I began to see that the business of life is to live, and to live well. In some ways, I still carried the emotional burden of my former life. I needed to be reborn. I needed a challenge, a goal, something to shoot for, but what? I was about to come face to face with the answer to that question—an answer that lay about 2000 miles away, spanned 15 miles across and was more than 4000 feet deep. It was time to revisit an old friend—and adversary.

Part Five
Rebirth

Chapter Fifteen

A Day in the Life Of a Fit Man

Twelve miles, 3000 feet, and the challenge of the Grand Canyon

Arizona's Grand Canyon is one of those rare places that somehow manages to be both unremarkable and unforgettable. In 1540, in an area somewhere near the northeastern border of what is now Arizona, the Spanish explorer Francisco Vasquez de Coronado dispatched a group of twelve men to follow up on the claims of their Hopi guides about the existence of a great canyon to the west. When they reached the canyon twenty days later, theirs were the first European eyes to cast across the great ocean of space. Despite what those eyes beheld, there was disbelief among the Spaniards regarding the actual size of the canyon, and so in the manner typical of reckless tourists, a plan was put forth to trek down to the thin sliver of blue that was the Colorado River, which the explorers took to be no more than six feet wide. Hours later, they returned, exhausted, having only made it one third of the way toward their goal before realizing the magnitude of their error in judgment. They had discovered what generations of future tourists would come to know; that it is the ability of the canyon to exceed the limits of human comprehension that make it so completely unforgettable.

Ever since then, generations of amateur and professional explorers still come, camera in hand, to faithfully document their experiences. Unlike the men of Coronado's time, these new explorers will return home with color photographs and digital video to back up their story. It is these innumerable millions of pictures framed within their five-by-seven borders of white or the wall calendars with postcard-perfect images that become "the canyon" in the minds of many. Our familiarity with these fleeting images is so deeply imbedded in our common memory that upon seeing the canyon for the first time, usually from the popular vantage point of the south rim, the effect, for some of us, is like looking at just another picture—larger, yes, but completely unremarkable.

When something as grand as the Grand Canyon becomes as blasé as a postcard, the only thing left to do is to venture beyond the rim. To descend into the embrace of these narrow walls of sepia hues is to "see" the canyon with much more than just your eyes. To feel the quickening pace of one's own heart, as mind and muscle rally against the inexorable forces of inertia and gravity on the long hike up, is to experience at a gut level what wind, water, and a little bit of time can accomplish.

The first time Mary and I ventured beyond the rim was on a clear morning in September, 1986. We had been married less than three months when we decided to make the trip. I was twenty-six years old at the time, and weighed somewhere in the neighborhood of 200 pounds. As a former weight lifter, I was strong and packed quite a bit of muscle. Mary was twenty-eight and lithe, with an astounding grace, the result of hours of yoga. We were both avid hikers, having spent many a weekend exploring trails from Arizona's arid deserts in the south to the cold mountains in the north. In those days, we favored a low-fat diet, along with plenty of exercise that included jogging, moderate weight training for me, and yoga. We were not very particular about where our food came from, and because we kept different schedules and were years away from being parents, we were especially fond of the convenience of processed foods.

It had not escaped my notice that despite my busy schedule and active life, I had steadily gained weight since college. A small "bicycle tire" of stored fat encircled my waist, and my pants size had enlarged somewhat. I didn't quite know what to make of these changes, as I was clearly not trying to gain weight. Like Boxer, the doomed horse in George

Chapter Fifteen: A Day in the Life Of a Fit Man

Orwell's *Animal Farm*, I believed the solution to my small but growing weight problem was to work harder. I was therefore increasingly determined to avoid fat in my diet and to exercise more.

Another perplexing feature of my health was that despite all the exercise—even in college when I was running four to twelve miles most days—I noticed that rather than feeling better, the exercise left me in pain. Even though I was trim and solidly muscled at six feet and 200 pounds, my legs ached miserably after a long run. I took this to be normal as I had experienced minor aches and pains after a hard workout for as long as I could remember. Along with the fatigue, I would often end a long run with a fitful and usually violent coughing spell. I didn't know it then, but I had asthma and it would only worsen over the years. In a stunning feat of irrational logic, I came to accept the aches and pains, respiratory problems, and fatigue as the price of being healthy.

The Grand Canyon stretches across the northern end of Arizona for 277 miles, averaging 4,000 feet deep with a 6,000 foot drop at its greatest depth. The widest point in the canyon spans 15 miles. The Bright Angel trail was built by the Havasupai Indians and served as their highway between the canyon rim and Indian Gardens below. The trail is rated as strenuous or difficult by most, and runs 12 miles round trip along the section we planned to hike from its starting point on the rim out to Plateau Point, six miles away. This section of the trail has an elevation change of more than 3000 feet, with sometimes dramatically changing temperatures between those extremes.

In 1986, we took the Bright Angel Trail down from the south rim, along a series of switchbacks that hugged the sheer walls of the canyon, out to our destination, a dramatic overlook called Plateau Point, which put us about fifteen hundred feet above the Colorado river.

Some experienced long-haul hikers and backpackers consider the Bright Angel trail to be one of the "easier" trails into the canyon. As you might expect, easy is a relative term when used in this context. Despite the fact that the trail is usually well populated and water is available at several locations, it is a grueling hike. The trip down, while deceptively easy at first, becomes quite the opposite by the time you get to the bottom. Some people refer to the canyon as an inverted mountain, because you climb down first, then climb back up. What you discover on the way down is that the pitch of the trail and the pull of gravity force you to walk in a crouched, bent-leg manner that ultimately wears out your knees and the sheath of muscles that make up the thigh. By the time we reached the four-and-a-half mile mark at an unlikely oasis of cottonwood trees and shaded camp sites called Indian Gardens, our legs were already wobbly from the trip down. We persevered the rest of the distance out to the plateau, where we stopped to rest and enjoy the view. Lunch was a bag of trail mix. It had been cold up on the rim, but down on the plateau, the weather was lovely.

We took some pictures and surveyed the river below, which was brown with sediment. We were in good spirits and spoke about the wonderful dinner we would have upon our triumphant return to the rim. After playing hide and seek with a squirrel, whic had apparently staked a claim on this prime piece of real estate, we finally packed our gear and headed back. The first mile and a half on the way back was fine as it was relatively flat, but once we passed through Indian Gardens and hit the steep trail, we began to experience Grand Canyon "hiker's remorse." The hike down seemed easy at first, but it had taken a toll on our legs. Now the four remaining miles up the steep cliffs would test us and test us they did. Before long, Mary, her body drained of vital minerals suffered severe muscle cramps in both legs. She could bear no more than ten paces without stopping to rest. I was doing fine for the first mile up, but soon I too began to grow weary.

The last mile or two was agony for both of us. We must have looked like accident victims to the sympathetic strangers who passed us. Many took pity and offered words of encouragement, but these fell on deaf ears. Every step felt as though it might be our last. At about a quarter mile from the top, my left leg cramped up so badly that I could not extend it completely. When we finally reached the rim, instead of celebrating as we planned, we shuffled off in the general direction of our cabin. We were in such a debilitated state that we were quite literally delirious, and could not remember where exactly our cabin was.

We stumbled around in the woods for what seemed like forever, until, quite by accident, I found the cabin. When I looked around, I noted that Mary was nowhere to be seen. The selfish instinct to survive had kicked in and I had abandoned her somewhere along the way. Eventually, she too found her way to the cabin.

The sun was still up, so it must have been somewhere around late afternoon when we arrived back. The odd thing is that neither of us has any recollection of what happened after we made it back. Apparently we showered and changed clothes, but we know this only because when we awoke the next morning, we were in our pajamas. Did we go to dinner as we had planned? Did we talk about our trip and revel in our victory? I don't know and neither does Mary. I ruled out alien abduction as a potential cause of the gaps in our memory, and accepted that the hike had essentially transformed us into walking zombies, exhausted beyond consciousness.

The next morning was Sunday, so we decided to attend a sunrise service held on the rim of the canyon. We should have been exultant at the realization of our dream, and at the transforming prospect of having Sunday service on the rim of the canyon as the sun breaks over the horizon. Instead, we were bundled up in every stitch of clothing we brought with us. While it was cold and it looked like it might snow, judging by the curious stares of onlookers, we were a lot colder than everyone else. Mary could barely walk, and shuffled along as if she were recovering from a long and debilitating illness. Her skin pallid, her eyes flat and lifeless, she had the wide eyed uncomprehending stare of a prisoner of war who has seen far too much. She mumbled more than spoke and looked as though she might fall over at any moment. I'm certain I didn't look any better.

I don't recall what happened after the service. Did we eat breakfast at one of the hotel restaurants? I can't say. All I do remember is getting into the car and driving past the morning activity on the rim. I have no memory of the five-hour trip home, some parts of which required navigating steep mountain roads, nor do I have any memory of anything else that happened for the remainder of that day.

To put it mildly, with the exception of the hike, we blacked out most of the rest of that trip. We were young and supposedly healthy, but the outcome of that trip in 1986 proved we had a lot to learn about what really constitutes good health. We vowed never to venture "below the rim" again. As the years progressed and our health declined, we became even more certain that we would never see the inner Canyon again. Though much of that trip has eroded from memory, I treasured what I could remember, because it was all either of us had, and as far as we were concerned, it was all we would ever have.

RETURN TO THE CANYON

It came as something of a surprise when the thought popped into my head to hike the Grand Canyon again. It was fall 2004, and I was rolling along on Washington DC's Beltway, Interstate 495, in the always-congested mid-morning rush hour traffic. I called Mary and said, "I want to hike the Canyon. It'll be fun and it'll prove that what we've accomplished with our health goes beyond just the window dressing of how we look. It'll prove that we really are stronger and healthier than we once were. Set it up."

Mary remembered enough of our last hike to pause a moment. Then she spoke. "Canyon, the Grand Canyon?" As accustomed to my out-of-left-field announcements as she was, this one startled her. I could hear the incredulity in her voice, but almost immediately, she followed up with a little laugh and an "OK." She knew the difference between when I was just talking to hear the sound of my own voice and when I really meant to follow through on something.

We talked about the trip and the hike later that evening and over the next few weeks. We settled on February 2005 as our target, which left us three months to prepare. There were the logistics to consider, and a half dozen reasons why we couldn't make the trip and shouldn't

Chapter Fifteen: A Day in the Life Of a Fit Man

attempt to hike the canyon. Among them were the weather, my asthma, the approximately 5,500 foot change in altitude from our home in Virginia to the Canyon's south rim, jet lag and restaurant food. In the end, all those excuses—and that is exactly what they were—could not stand against the irresistible pull of the Canyon.

One of the issues I had to deal with was my asthma. We would be visiting friends and family in Phoenix three days before our hike. Phoenix is dry and dusty, and contrary to the myth of the desert as a refuge for asthmatics, it is the exact opposite. The last time I visited Phoenix was in January of 2002. I was only in town for three days, but during that time, my asthma degenerated from an intermittent cough to a violent series of attacks. After I returned home, it was several weeks before the symptoms subsided completely. How, I wondered, would I survive two-and-a-half days of breathing the air in Phoenix? Would my asthma symptoms, which had completely disappeared after I changed my diet, return and prevent me from hiking the Canyon?

A second issue was weather. The prospect of hiking Bright Angel trail in winter seemed, well, slightly crazy to us. Just getting to the canyon on northern Arizona's icy roads, which sometimes required tire chains, was a frightening proposition. It took great effort on my part to dispel the unpleasant images of our car stuck on a lonely side road in a snow drift, or the sickening feeling that comes from slipping on a narrow icy ledge and disappearing over the edge of a cliff in a snow storm.

During the two weeks leading up to our trip, the weather forecasts for the canyon played on our emotions, alternating between bright and sunny to cold and snowy. We were in Phoenix when the "final" forecast, two days before the hike, forecast snow on the Monday we planned for our great adventure. One good omen was the fact that I passed the asthma test. I was starting to have second thoughts about the snow, but Mary reminded me about why we made the trip and so, on a brisk Sunday morning—Mary, the girls and myself—found ourselves heading north along Arizona Interstate 17. The weather forecast had not improved. It was worse, in fact, predicting snowfall beginning Sunday night rather than Monday morning. We wanted to be in our hotel before the storm, so except for a stop in Flagstaff to buy crampons (spikes) for our boots, we did not delay.

Clouds had been building on the northern horizon on the trip up and continued to do so all the way to the Canyon. By the time we checked into our hotel, the sky had the unmistakable look of an impending storm. Snow and ice still covered much of the ground from a previous storm. Despite the coming weather and the stinging chill in the air, I couldn't help noticing how different the south rim is in winter. Gone are the crowds of summer, the jarring chorus of a dozen languages of visitors from all over the world. In winter, one can almost imagine the Canyon as it might have been when Coronado's men first ventured there. Of course, winter also means fewer people on the trail who can help when things don't go as planned.

The El Tovar, the grandest of the south rim hotels, was closed for renovations. I had hoped to stand before the great fireplace in her lobby and be encouraged for the task ahead by its warmth. There was little warmth to be had now. The hotel, in gloomy earthen tones, stood cold and empty against the encroaching snow and a darkening sky. It reminded me of the famous and dreadful Overlook Hotel from Stephen King's novel, *The Shining*. I couldn't ignore the fact that King's story unfolded in winter as well.

The view of the hotel was depressing, but the views of the Canyon were spectacular. I looked out over the rim as my eyes tracked the trail all the way out to Plateau Point. Our destination seemed farther than it had been 18 years ago. I went to bed that night with more than a bit of apprehension about the coming day.

4:30am

I awoke early. It was too dark outside to tell whether any snow had fallen, but the cold air off the frosted window pane told me that it had. The Weather Channel replayed the depressing details of the day ahead. The prediction now was only for snow flurries throughout the day, but that meant that it would be cold, with wind chills in the lower

20s. This also meant that there would be ice on the trail. I did not relish the idea of descending into the canyon along the steep and narrow trail on a sheet of ice. Add snow at the upper levels near the rim, and rain beneath the snow line as we trekked deeper into the canyon, and you had the recipe for difficulties far surpassing those of our last hike 18 years ago, when we were younger and presumably stronger. I began to wonder whether we were not getting in over our heads. Soon Mary and the girls were awake and dressed.

6:30am

We decided to get breakfast at the Bright Angel lodge. It was still dark, but the crunch of fresh snow beneath our boots provided further evidence of the snow that fell overnight. The menu at the restaurant had a so-called "hiker's" breakfast that included cold cereal, fruit, and a muffin—a grain and sugar recipe for getting stranded at the bottom. Instead, we had eggs cooked in butter with a side of bacon. Mary wanted a breakfast steak, but the only steak on the menu was chicken fried. The waiter acknowledged that the steaks came pre-made and that there was no way to separate the batter from the steak. So much for real cooking.

We rounded off our breakfast with a healthy dose of unrefined coconut oil, which we brought from home. We also stashed away a second helping in the amount of several tablespoons in small plastic-lidded cups which we intended to use once we were on the trail. The coconut oil had hardened to a stiff consistency in the cold climate. I broke off a portion and popped it into my mouth. It had the mouth feel of crunchy candy without any of the redeeming qualities of candy. Though I don't relish the taste of straight coconut oil, I've come to appreciate its appetite-suppressing, energy-boosting, and well-being-inducing properties, so I ate it gladly.

After breakfast, I found a wide-brimmed hat in the gift shop, which was more suitable to wet weather than the knit cap I had brought along. As we walked back to our room to get our gear, there was enough light now to see the canyon. To our amazement, it was no longer there. In its place was a sea of clouds that seemed to stretch all the way to the north rim, a sight both beautiful and frightening. Mary and I grew up in the central deserts of Arizona. We were well accustomed to triple digit temperatures that made it hot enough to poach an egg on the hood of your car, but snow, ice and freezing temperatures were a bit beyond our experience. Above us, a second cloud ceiling sent light snow falling. We were both in a hurry to get going. To stop and think too much about the conditions was to invite doubt and perhaps even failure. We were prepared. We had water, warm clothing, sturdy boots, ski poles and crampons for negotiating the icy trail. Once we were geared up, it would have been easy to mistake us for experienced winter hikers.

7:30am

We returned to our room, geared up and gave final instructions to Stephanie and Raven. They would be staying topside, awaiting our return. Stephanie slumped at the edge of the bed, her posture a study in despondency. I can only imagine what was going through her mind. She had grown up in a sheltered suburban cocoon, far from the fickle whims of Mother Nature. It must have seemed to her that we were embarking on an Everest-like expedition where neither success nor life was guaranteed.

The immensity of the canyon and the larger than life drama of the storm made her fearful. I explained that the snow would dissipate once we descended below the snow line, but I could see that for the moment, she longed for the parents she knew when she was younger, the doddering, overweight, TV-watching parents, who could always be found on the sofa, always made safe, sensible decisions and never took chances. I reminded her that we were the same parents she had always known. We might be thinner and more adventurous, but we knew how to handle ourselves in the outdoors. As I offered these words of comfort, I tried to believe them myself.

We left the room and walked the short distance to the Bright Angel trailhead behind the Kolbe Studio building, which perched precariously at the rim of the canyon. We put on our crampons and headed down the trail.

Chapter Fifteen: A Day in the Life Of a Fit Man

. . . .

8:30am

The Bright Angel trail is made up of a series of short switchback "steps" that zigzag along the canyon walls in the steepest sections of the trail. Opposite the wall, the trail terminates in a cliff which drops off abruptly into the abyss. Switchbacks can make the trail seem longer than it needs to be, but without them, the trail would be prohibitively steep. We cautiously made our way down, using our hiking poles to maintain our balance, and took extra care to dig our crampons into the ice.

To our surprise, we saw tracks in the snow ahead of us. The deeply etched boot prints told us there were two of them and though out of sight, they were not far ahead. It was reassuring to see that someone else thought it was a good idea to go for a walk on a morning like this. Maybe we weren't crazy after all.

The going was dicey at first. Once we got over the initial excitement of finally being on the trail, we had to get used to walking with crampons on the steep downhill slope while not getting disoriented by the swirling snow and the stinging cold. While we walked, we talked and took care to follow the tracks ahead of us. Sometimes they hugged the rock face side of the trail. At other times, the tracks veered dangerously close to the cliff edge. Visibility was extremely poor in the heavy mist and flying snow. I reminded myself that we could turn back anytime if the conditions worsened. At the same time, I couldn't help thinking that if we could just make it below the snow line, we would be fine.

On the upper trail, the route passes through two narrow arched tunnels, cut out of the canyon sandstone. On a descent, the first tunnel is a relatively short distance from the start of the trail. The second, slightly larger tunnel is where we caught up with the two hikers ahead of us. They were a tall man in his mid to late twenties and a shorter, much older man who could have been in his sixties. They might have been father and son. This is an amazing thing about the Canyon—you meet such a diverse group of people when you venture below the rim. When you see someone who bests you by more than twenty years on the trail, it makes it all the more difficult to complain about how hard the hike is. We've encountered many older people on the Arizona trails we've hiked over the years. Our dream has always been to become that "older couple in their sixties," scruffy and muddy, with wide grins that inspire the "kids" in their twenties and thirties to, as Mary's mom likes to say, "just keep on livin.'" We bid our fellow hikers goodbye and left them to the shelter of the tunnel.

As we continued on the trail, the snow lessened and the mist began to lift. The temperature shifted a few degrees warmer and brought intermittent bouts of sleet. There were icy sections of the trail that required careful placement of each step to ensure the crampons bit deeply enough to prevent slips. Eventually, the ice and snow gave way to a frozen sludge, and we could see farther now as the mist lifted and the canyon came slowly into focus, like a black and white photo in a bath of developer. The toughest part of the hike was finally over, we thought. We were wrong.

We were beneath the low hanging clouds that concealed the canyon from viewers on the rim. The snow, now turned into a light rain, tapped gently on the brim of my hat. The rain was a welcome sign that marked the end of the ice. Unfortunately, it also turned the normally dusty canyon trail into a river of mud. Our crampons were of little use at this stage. We found walking down-slope in mud to be a particularly tricky maneuver. Every third step or so, our feet would slide in the slippery goo. Step, step, slide, step, step, slide; it went on like this for some time over a series of steep switchbacks known as Jacob's Ladder. Though we had experienced similar terrain in the forested mountains of Hawaii many years ago, this was uniquely different. What made it different, and worse, were the mules.

Practically every day of the year, a mule train made up of six or more mules makes its way down the trail behind a rough-and-ready guide who typically looks like an extra from a western movie. Each mule carries one tourist who, depending on their ability to handle heights, is either frightened or delighted. For those people who don't want to or can't walk the trail, the mule train is a great way to see the inner canyon. The rules of the trail dictate that the mules have right of way. When a mule train approaches, hikers are advised to stand quietly by the side of the trail and let them pass.

The mules we encountered were heading down-trail as we were. We stood aside and nodded toward each mule and its rider as they passed. After they passed, the trail, which had been difficult to traverse before, was almost impossible now. The combined weight of the mules and their riders gouged great hoofed holes, several inches deep, into the mud. The mules also defecated as they walked. The dark green, steamy piles of mule-flop were ground into the mud by the next mule in line, turning the trail into a kind of sticky, stinking, boot-sucking mud pudding. Now, not only did we have to take care not to misstep, slip and go careening off a cliff, but we also had to make certain not to step in any "green" mud as well. As a final insult, the trail now reeked with the roadside grenades.

Just as I was beginning to think it might be best to turn around, the rain lessened and the stickiness of the mud subsided. We were on the lower levels of the trail above Indian Gardens, about three quarters of the way along our journey. Though much drier, the trail was littered with tennis ball-sized rocks eager to help me twist my ankle.

10:45am

We caught up with the mule train at Indian Gardens, where they stopped to tie up and give the riders a chance to regain some feeling in their rear ends. Indian Gardens is a lovely spot for a hiker to take a break before heading on to the river or out to Plateau Point. The Gardens get their name from their original inhabitants, the Havasupai Indians, who raised corn and beans here as late as the early 1900s. A small creek flows through this area making it a tranquil and refreshing sanctuary.

Mary and I decided not to stop here and pressed on instead. The trail to Plateau Point continues on for another mile and a half, where it ends at a dramatic bluff that overlooks the turbulent Colorado River, 1,500 feet below. The terrain between the Gardens and the Point is relatively flat and makes for an easy, almost relaxing walk. We wanted to get there before the mule train, so we had little time for strolling, and yet, the beauty of the Canyon from this vantage point could not be ignored. The ground was carpeted in desert greenery thanks to an extraordinary amount of rain in the past month or so. We saw the strangest cacti, dressed in brilliant purple colors, along the trail. The canyon walls rose up around us until they seemed to touch the sky. Above us, the cloud ceiling had broken up, revealing a brilliant blue canopy.

11:15am

·I was first to reach Plateau Point, but quickly discovered I was not alone. I walked to the edge of the rocky ledge to get a better view of the inner canyon and was surprised by the sight of a great black California condor resting on a lower ledge. The bird unfolded its wings to about half mast, a sight that took the breath right out of me. Never had I been this close to a condor outside of a zoo. The experience was incredible. Mary and the riders from the mule train soon joined me on the ledge where we all sat down for lunch. The bad weather had abated, turning what had been an inauspicious morning into a perfect day. We had made it to the halfway point of our journey. Neither snow, sleet nor rain had stayed us from our destination. All that remained was getting back up to the rim. For now, though, it was time to relax and enjoy our accomplishment.

In 1986, at this very same spot, we had enjoyed a bag of trail mix for lunch. We would not repeat that mistake again. We needed a mixture of energy in the form of slow-burning carbohydrates, protein and even slower-burning fat to fuel our return trip, so our lunch included home made beef jerky, a banana, some salted almonds (which we soaked and dehydrated prior to the trip), and a second dose of coconut oil. We washed our meal down with water, then took some pictures and enjoyed the view.

It was a bit hard for us to grasp the significance of where we were. Little more than a year-and-a-half earlier, the only way either of us would have been able to make it to Plateau Point would have been by helicopter.

Chapter Fifteen: A Day in the Life Of a Fit Man

. . . .

In those days, we both exceeded the 200 pound weight limit set for the mules. In my own case, I exceeded that number by an additional 200 pounds at least. Standing there with the Colorado River churning below, we celebrated this great accomplishment of rebirth and renewal.

The wind picked up some, and we both noticed how cold we had become. The clouds were regrouping above us, and we had several hours of up-canyon hiking ahead of us before we could mark this work completed. It was time to go. We said goodbye to our new friends from the mule train, geared up and headed back up the trail.

11:45am

The trip back to Indian Gardens passed quickly, but about a half mile from the shelter of the Gardens, the storm mounted its second assault. It began with a light rain that suddenly turned into hail. This was most unexpected. Weather down in the canyon is generally milder, but here we were being pelted with small stones of ice. Growing up in Arizona, we knew that hailstorms in the desert were often followed by torrential rains. We quickened our pace. A loud siren went off up ahead in the direction of the Gardens. It was a bit disorienting to hear this mechanical noise amidst sounds of nature. By now, the hail had turned into rain, which steadily grew in intensity. As we drew near the Gardens, I looked over my shoulder to see whether I could spot the mule train which had left the plateau shortly after we did. What I saw instead was a wall of water stretching from the heavens to the bottom of the canyon below. A celestial waterfall roared from the sky, practically obliterating the view behind us. I felt sorry for the mule riders. We had reached the relative safety of a covered information kiosk at the Gardens, but they were still out there. We decided to take a break at the Gardens and see how the storm would play out.

At the time, I didn't know that four-and-a-half miles away, and about 3000 vertical feet above us, the south rim of the Grand Canyon was under siege. Snow poured down from the heavens with the singular purpose of burying everything in sight. A bitter wind whipped the snow into a dancing fury until it seemed as though it was snowing from four different directions at once. If we had foreseen this, we would never have left our hotel room.

In fact, at that moment, Stephanie was looking out the window and wondering what had become of us. At 14 years old, she was the big sister, left in charge while we were away. At the height of the storm, a shrill siren pierced the air and made heads turn in the lobby of the Bright Angel hotel. Stephanie didn't know what the siren meant, but suspected it wasn't good. As Raven prepared for lunch from our store of food, Stephanie pulled the curtains and tried to shut out the cry of the storm.

12:15pm

In the Canyon, the rain finally began to let up. I sought shelter beneath a covered picnic table while Mary made her way back from the rest room. The mule train pulled into Indian Gardens, thoroughly soaked, at about the same time Mary left the rest room. She struck up a conversation with one of the riders. The trail guide had heard a loud boom preceding the siren, and was checking, via walkie-talkie, to find out what the trail conditions were. Less than a month ago, torrential rains had caused a landslide along the upper reaches of the trail, shutting the route down for a time while repairs were made. The prospect of being marooned, even in such a beautiful place as the Canyon, while a storm raged above us on the rim, was more than either of us could bear. Our children were up there. Landslide or not, we weren't going to stick around to find out whether the trail was still intact. We stayed just long enough for Mary to wrap her right knee with medical tape in preparation for the hike up. We checked our gear and set off once again.

12:30pm

As we started out along the rocky trail that lay beyond Indian Gardens, I let Mary take the lead. Her more deliberate pace would ensure that I wouldn't go too fast in the early phase of the return trip and burn myself out. On our 1986 hike, my legs were already shaky from the trip down. Now, although I felt a bit tired, my legs were only slightly fatigued. This was good news, but not the best news I could imagine, because the hardest, steepest part of the trail was still far ahead of us.

Chapter Fifteen: A Day in the Life Of a Fit Man

. . . .

My breathing was a different issue. As we made our way uphill, my breaths came in ragged spurts. I would never make it to the top like this, I realized, so I focused on the early morning wind sprints I ran, in the dark, on the hills back home in Virginia when the temperatures were in the 20s. I reminded myself of "suicide hill," that punishing incline along our favorite bike path that took me several tries before I could make it to the top without losing a lung along the way. Pretty soon, my breathing evened out as Indian Gardens fell further behind with each step.

The mule train left Indian Gardens shortly after we did, and so it wasn't long before they caught up with us. We stepped aside and found a couple of suitable rocks to sit on, thankful for the opportunity to rest our feet. I was feeling more tired now and knew that I was in for a challenge. After the mules passed, we picked up and followed them.

It was at this point that I made an amazing discovery. My legs, which had been feeling slightly fatigued earlier, now felt remarkably fresh. What's more, my breathing was calm, and to my surprise, I felt unexpectedly energized. I couldn't believe that a paltry two minutes of rest had reinvigorated me to this degree, but then I remembered the coconut oil. I knew that those medium-chain saturated fats in coconut oil were healthy, and provided long-burning energy for difficult workouts, but here I was experiencing the effect in one of nature's most divine laboratories. I expected my new-found energy to dissipate quickly, as it often did after a short rest on a long hike, but this time it didn't. Like the Energizer bunny, I kept going and going and going. I felt as if I could walk to the canyon rim and keep on going, all the way back home to Virginia if I wanted to. I thought about all the times in the past when I had "carbo-loaded" prior to a run or a workout, thought about the 10K race I ran years ago, and how I ran out of steam halfway through. I had loaded up on carbohydrates for that race while dutifully making sure I avoided as much fat as possible. How could so many people be so wrong about what the human body needs? How, and perhaps more important, why, did we lose our way?

As important as these questions were, Mary and I had a more pressing issue to deal with, namely, making it back to the rim. We pushed on, stopping now and then to rest or whenever the mule train about 50 yards ahead of us stopped for the guide to deliver some bit of Grand Canyon lore. It wasn't long before we encountered the mud again. The rain had stopped and we discovered it's easier to walk uphill in mud than downhill. Still, the mud which caked on our boots slowed our pace. Each step, in fact, required more energy output and exerted an extra amount of strain on our weary muscles than if we had been hiking up a dry trail and the trail was particularly steep in some places along this section.

The nice thing about having reached your destination somewhere within the Canyon is that you have no choice but to climb back out, no matter how tired you might be. Mary and I were finally starting to feel the strain of the hike, but we had plenty of energy left to return us to that part of the trail that was layered with snow. The temperature had warmed the ground sufficiently to turn the ice at the lower level of this section into frozen slush. Hiking uphill makes balancing oneself a bit easier, so we didn't bother putting our crampons back on.

Although the ground was apparently warmer, we seemed colder, especially when we stopped to rest, and resting was happening with greater frequency now. Although we had taken great care to find the right boots for the hike, we were less careful in the choice of clothing we wore. We made the grievous error of wearing cotton and cotton blend clothing beneath our waterproof outer jackets. Inside my jacket, I was sweating like a fountain. Down below in the canyon, this wasn't much of a problem, but in the cold air above the snow line this was a potentially dangerous combination of errors. We were still at least an hour from the rim and the comfort of a warm room and hot shower. By wearing cotton close to our skin, we had exposed ourselves to hypothermia and inadvertently violated one of the cardinal caveats of winter hiking: cotton kills. I didn't realize how wet I was, but every time we stopped to rest along the steep icy trail, I grew steadily colder. Mary's hands had become chilled in the frigid air.

Every turn at every switchback seemed like it would be the one where we would see some clue that we were close to the top. As we rounded each switchback, I kept expecting to see the arched tunnel that we passed through on the way down. If I didn't know any better, I would have sworn that someone had moved it. Although we could see the rim and even people at a distance, it seemed that with each step, the rim receded an equal distance away. Finally, the tunnel appeared. I almost shouted when I saw it. We were closing in on the end of our journey, but we were also colder and weaker.

Our pace was practically geriatric now. It wasn't that we were exhausted, rather we were taking our time, conserving our energy for the final push up the last hill. We knew that even though we were close, we still had some distance to cover. These last steps were the most difficult. It is a fact of human experience that the closer one comes to reaching one's goals, the more obstacles get in the way. The first tunnel appeared before us and then it was behind us. We could see the Kolbe Studio building a short distance in front of us. We walked the last few switchbacks and emerged, finally, at the top of the trail and the end of our journey.

There was no marching band, no cheering crowds and barely a single person to welcome us. We hugged for a moment and then kissed. We stared at each other for a long while, our faces streaked with rain and our clothes wet and covered with mud and dirt. We looked awful, but that didn't stop us from laughing loud and long. We may have looked like two bits on the outside, but at that moment we felt like a million dollars inside.

As we walked back to our room we were jubilant. We stopped for a moment at a vantage point along the rim where we had stood the day before and gazed out at the trail, six miles long and over 3000 feet deep. Even now, it was hard to believe we had actually done it.

A Life Unburdened

. . . .

Richard and Mary at Plateau Point in the Grand Canyon, 2005

We took our time traversing the paved icy walkways around the Bright Angel Lodge. Our route took us up a flight of steps and down a long, narrow outside walkway. I was beyond discomfort at this point and simply longed to see my daughters. When we reached our room, I gave the door a loud pounding. "Pizza delivery!" The door opened and Stephanie and Raven exploded from the room and smothered us in excited hugs. It was good to be "home."

Less than two years earlier, we existed in a crisis state of obesity, high blood pressure, asthma, chronic pain, depression, weakened immune systems and a sense of hopelessness about the direction our lives had taken. A mere nineteen months later, we were hiking the Grand Canyon. We now know, without a shred of doubt, that there are no limits to what a willing heart, an active mind and yes, lots of good food, can accomplish. With this defining challenge behind us, we were finally free to live a life unburdened.

Chapter Sixteen

Ten Steps To A New Life

Food is key, but recreating your life involves more than just what you eat

Think about the last time you were successful at something. It may have involved achieving an important goal at work or school, or perhaps you landed your dream job or forged a promising new relationship. To achieve this goal, you probably executed some sort of plan. Even if you weren't entirely conscious of a plan, when you review the steps you took to successfully reach your goal, the plan you used begins to emerge.

There's an old saying: "If you fail to plan, you plan to fail." It's true. When you attempt to reach an objective without a clear plan, it is very much like trying to find an address in an unfamiliar city without any directions. While you might stumble upon your destination, it's much more likely that you'll remain lost. Even with a plan sometimes, if it is not the right plan for you, success may prove elusive.

This is how it was with me for years, as I bounced from diet to diet. I followed one plan after another, and encountered defeat in every instance. I eventually realized that I needed to take a more proactive role by designing a plan that worked for me, rather than blindly following someone else's plan. This is much easier to do than it sounds. To begin with, you don't have to start from scratch. I didn't. I discovered over the years that even though there was no one perfect weight loss and fitness plan for me, there were many plans that incorporated methods that did work for me. The trick was in identifying those parts of a plan that worked, and knowing which parts to discard.

When I was a vegetarian, I found that a plant-based diet did not work for me, but in the process of making this discovery I learned a valuable lesson about the importance of buying in-season produce. When I tried low-carbohydrate dieting, I realized right away that this approach to nutrition was incompatible with me as well, but I also discovered a critical need to limit sugar in my diet. In time, I was able to devise an approach to nutrition and exercise that was tailored to my life. You can do the same with a little bit of work. You'll discover that just like a tailored suit, a tailored plan for health and fitness will fit you much better, and last longer than an "off the rack" solution.

Typically, books on diet, weight loss and fitness tend to focus on recipes and exercise routines. These are important components of a successful health improvement plan, but they are not the only components that should be considered. One of the most important things Mary and I discovered on our journey was that improving our health required a multidisciplinary approach that went far beyond nutrition and exercise. The ten steps listed in an earlier chapter are the same ten steps we used to improve our lives. Here they are again in a slightly different format.

1. Educate yourself.
2. Match the size of the commitment to the size of the problem.
3. Rely on the strength of your tribe.
4. Create harmony in your life.
5. Simplify your life.
6. Eat as if your life depended on it.
7. Make exercise a part of your life.
8. Get plenty of high quality sleep.
9. Find your motivation.
10. Share what you've learned.

Step 1: Educate yourself

Every successful human endeavor began with a question. Whether it was the discovery of the practical application of fire as a tool for cooking or the landing of a remote explorer on the moon of a distant planet, every accomplishment in the history of humankind began with a single question, fueled by curiosity. This need to know and understand the world around us leads to the acquisition of knowledge, and ultimately, the discovery of truth.

With our busy, modern lives and our insatiable need for instant gratification, we rarely ask questions anymore, relying instead on others to do the work of uncovering the truth. Much like our agricultural ancestors, who forsook the independence of their hunter/gatherer lives for the stability of communal life, we too have come to depend on the "village" experts to ask the questions and provide the sustenance that makes possible our very existence. Our nutritional experts come as a diverse collection of doctors, nutritionists, dieticians, food producers and government bureaucrats. Dependence upon these professionals to guide us in making the right decisions about our health is not inherently wrong, but given the sorry state of personal health and fitness in America today, one cannot help but wonder whether the experts are really up to the job.

In times like these, a stiff spine and a frontiersman's penchant for "doing it yourself" is just what's needed. That's what this first of ten steps is about: asking questions and finding your own answers. It's for the professionals to debate the issues, write position papers and attend scholarly conferences in sunny locales to discuss "the obesity problem," but we've got living to do today, and need practical answers and actionable information now, so let's get on with it.

THE SEARCH FOR KNOWLEDGE

Walk into any bookstore or library and make your way to the diet section. There you'll find hundreds of books on weight management and health. Never let it be said that we are not a health-conscious people.

A Life Unburdened

· ·

The ever-increasing number of books on the subject of weight loss is a testament to the interest we all have in improving our health and our lives. And let's not forget the Internet with its gigabits of dieting information available at the click of a button. You would think with so much information available few people would succumb to a weight problem and the illnesses that go with it, yet as a nation we are sicker than we've ever been. Cancer, heart disease and obesity-related illnesses continue to top the charts as our most popular ways to die. The profitability of the pharmaceutical industry, and the rise in weight-related adult disorders like Type 2 diabetes in children, is further evidence of the declining state of health in America.

Why then, with such an abundance of information at our fingertips, have we not been able to stem the tide of obesity and ill health? There is a line from the book of Hosea, in the Bible that says, "My people perish for lack of knowledge." This quote is irrefutable, for it is a lack of knowledge that condemns many of us to a fate of illness and disease. It was a lack of knowledge that almost did me in not long ago.

GETTING PAST "I KNOW."

One of the first things I had to get over was the idea that I already knew everything there was to know about nutrition. Even now, when I talk to people about the importance of learning, really learning, about nutrition and their own bodies, the inevitable reply is, "Yes, yes, I know all that, but just tell me what to eat."

My reply, when I'm feeling feisty is, "Do you really know?" I'll ask them if they know the difference between long-chain and short-chain fatty acids and how these fats are metabolized in the body. I'll ask them if they've ever heard of the Framingham Heart Study and how it has been used to both defend and discredit the cholesterol theory of heart disease which has been the principal influence behind our present-day dietary policy. I'll ask for their opinion on the merits of grass-fed versus grain-fed beef or what they know about the medicinal value of fermented foods, or even where do they stand on the issue of the enteric nervous system as the body's second "brain."

I almost always get blank stares when I ask these questions. I make it clear that my goal is not to belittle, but to point out that the body of knowledge regarding human nutrition does not exist in a vacuum, that it is a complex issue, and that like most complex issues, our understanding of it has been colored by political and economic concerns, which often supercede health concerns.

Only when I admitted that I didn't know as much as I thought I knew could I start on my quest to discover, for myself, what kind of dietary regimen worked best for me.

TAKING CHARGE

So what did I do? First, I learned about the foods I was eating. I asked the kinds of questions that were relevant to me, then went in search of answers. What was the composition of the foods I ate? How did they affect my body and my mind? How did my enteric nervous system power my gastrointestinal system? How did that system work? What were the different kinds of fats and carbohydrates, and how were they metabolized? What benefits were derived from dietary fat? Was saturated fat really bad for me? Was cholesterol bad or did it provide a useful function in the body? Why is it that after eating a large meal, I'm hungry again two hours later? Why didn't I have the energy to exercise? When I did exercise, why did I get tired so quickly? Which foods should I eat? Which foods should I cut back on? Which foods should I eliminate from my diet altogether? Why are soy and corn syrup included in so many convenience food products? How has government nutrition policy been affected by politics and economics? What influence do the food and pharmaceutical industries have on what I eat? Why isn't my doctor telling me more? How much of what I know or think I know about nutrition, weight loss and processed food is true?

INFORMATION RESOURCES

Information, and lots of it, is the real key to success. A plan and tools without the knowledge of their proper use are useless. You've got to know—I mean really know—why you're following a particular course. Knowledge really is power. If you're simply following some diet guru's advice you will probably fail in your efforts because blind obedience never lasts long. Real motivation and progress come from knowing about nutrition and fitness and what they mean to you personally, so you absolutely must read, think and learn. Some key places where you can find information are as follows:

THE INTERNET

Sure, there's lots of mindless drivel on the Internet, but there's also a gold mine of useful information on health and nutrition. It's hard to imagine that only a decade or so ago, this vast wealth of information did not exist for most people. Whether it's access to medical studies or the rants of real people who've had their stomachs stapled, the Internet is a boundless archive that puts information at your fingertips.

LIBRARIES

Don't overlook the public library. They haven't gone out of fashion just yet. One downside of the Internet is that there's no kindly bespectacled matron to help you find what you need. Libraries are wonderful places to get your hands on medical journals, for example, without having to pay the fees that similar access on the Internet might cost. Your local library may also provide free music rentals to give you something to do besides eat while you're driving home in rush hour traffic. You can also pick up exercise video tapes and DVDs at the library or, if like me you've got a thing for salsa (the dance, as well as the condiment), you can check out how-to videos as well. Who says exercise can't be fun? Libraries also host frequent book sales, so there's always an opportunity to pick up something on nutrition, exercise, and health at super cheap prices.

BOOKSTORES

Many bookstores have a bargain table where books have been drastically marked down. Here you can find great deals on health-oriented books. Remember, not everything you read is true or true for you, so be discriminating in your choices. That's where the thinking part comes in. I find it helpful to read opposing viewpoints on a particular subject. That's why reading and gathering information from a variety of resources is so important. If you're only getting one side of the story, you can't make an educated decision.

MAGAZINES AND NEWSPAPERS

Magazines and newspapers can be useful sources of information too, but be careful here, as many of these publications are supported by corporate largesse in the form of advertising. The result is that the editorial position of some newspapers and health magazines has become hopelessly contaminated through their economic dependence on corporate support. A good example of corporate contamination in action is a popular fitness magazine that had, in one issue, an extensive article on the "healthiest" prepared foods. Page after page of highly processed convenience foods were accompanied by rosy recommendations from a panel of nutrition "experts." Amazed, I wondered what kind of nutrition "expert" believes a candy bar is healthy? A little investigation revealed that all but one of the experts was a dietician.

The American Dietetic Association receives funding from a number of food industry interests. Even a casual review of their positions on food and nutrition reveals an organization that espouses a philosophy so close to that of the food industry that it is difficult to tell where one ends and the other begins.

TELEVISION

Television as a source of reliable health information should be regarded with the highest level of skepticism. In *The Truth about the Drug Companies*, Marcia Angell, M.D. reveals that a novel technique for consumer manipulation is to employ celebrities to inject pharmaceutical ads into what appears to be a casual, televised conversation. A medium so lacking in ethics that it would condone this type of manipulative marketing should be viewed with the most jaundiced of eyes.

Knowledge is just the beginning. Once you begin to understand the basic nuts and bolts of nutrition, exercise, and how your own body works, it's time to make a commitment to change. Is a vegetarian diet right for you? What about grass-fed beef, raw milk or fermented vegetables? You'll never know for sure unless you read, think, learn, and explore for yourself.

I believe the secret to improving your health is understanding that no one can do it for you but you . . . . and you can do it! As long as we depend on others (including our doctors) to "tell us what to do," we will never make meaningful progress toward our goals.

Step 2: Match the size of the commitment to the size of the problem

For years, Mary and I purchased one piece of exercise equipment after another. More often than not, that equipment spent more time as a clothes rack than a workout partner. When we finally made the commitment to build an in-home gym, we went all the way. We invested our money and our time. We integrated the gym into an overall wellness plan that included diet, improving our relationship and finances, and the pursuit of career goals—including my goal to become a public speaker.

Making commitments is easy. Sticking to them is work because real progress requires real commitment. This is why I believe that sometimes the "small steps" philosophy doesn't work, because it's difficult to take on a big challenge with a small solution. I believe you should think big and devise big solutions to solve big problems. Think big when you make your plan, but then execute that plan incrementally— in small steps. But isn't that the same thing as the small steps philosophy? No. Let me give you an example.

Chapter Sixteen: Ten Steps To A New Life

Saying you're going to take the stairs to your office instead of the elevator is a small step which, for many of us, results in failure. How many times have you taken a small step toward improving your health by buying a diet book, ordering a diet soda or signing up for the free trial period at your local gym? How many times did these small steps help you achieve your long-term goals?

The "problem" is that humans are task-oriented creatures, motivated by a powerful inner desire to meet the challenge of long-term goal achievement. Those achievements can be anything from getting rich to finding love to building a business or helping the poor. Isolated tasks with vaguely defined end-goals are like orphaned dreams. They disappear once we wake up and have to deal with the real world. So how do we achieve our important goals?

A better approach is to say "I want to enrich my life, so I'm going to climb Mount Kilimanjaro in Africa next year. To accomplish this goal, I'm going to improve my health and my diet by eating more whole foods, starting today. I'm going to study up on Tanzania, its culture and people, and I'm going to get a passport. Next weekend, I'm going to develop a plan that includes meals and exercise with goals set for the next 12 months, and the first step in my plan is that I'm going to take the stairs to my office every day, starting today." What a powerful commitment that is! As part of a master plan, the "baby steps" approach is a great strategy.

Without a long-term goal, a small step becomes an isolated step, unsupported by either a plan or a commitment. But a real goal is a powerful catalyst that lays the foundation for success. Instead of an isolated event with a high potential for failure, taking the stairs becomes a link in a chain of forward-moving events that speed you toward your goal.

I believe the major failing of the small steps approach is that it presumes failure in advance, and attempts to counter that potential for failure by reducing risk through the adoption of an approach built upon minimal effort. Goal achievers would call this planning to fail. Dream big, plan big, commit big, then execute—in small steps.

Step 3: Rely on the strength of your tribe

The concept of the tribe—a band of like-minded individuals united toward a common goal—is an old and established artifact of human behavior. From the tribe we both derive and lend support when needed. When we are trying to overcome a health crisis like obesity, we can look to our tribe of friends, family members and medical professionals for help.

I read an article a few years ago about a well-known gentleman in the public sphere who underwent a dramatic physical change. He was an extremely "stout" fellow, as they used to say, and I saw in him a kindred spirit who must surely understand the burden that I bore daily. Gastric bypass surgery was not the rage then as it is today, so this gentleman decided to lose weight the old-fashioned way, through diet and exercise. As a man of means, this fellow enjoyed the twin luxuries of a personal trainer and a personal chef. I was happy for him, if not a bit envious. I reasoned that losing weight must surely be a lot easier for someone who has a staff of professionals at his beck and call. I relied on this crutch of an excuse for years afterward, but eventually I had to face up to the fact that even if there was not another living soul on the planet on whom I could rely on for help, my health was still *my* problem and *my* responsibility.

Step three of our ten step plan is all about finding the help you need to reach your goals, even if that help begins and ends with just you. The inspiration for this step came, in part, from a dear friend who has her own problems with weight. She is a single woman of middle age and possessed of a cheerful spirit that can brighten any room. Upon congratulating my wife and me on our success, my friend remarked rather darkly that "it's different when you've got someone to help you." Her comment struck a chord and reminded me of my own similar observation years earlier about the aforementioned gentleman of means.

Chapter Sixteen: Ten Steps To A New Life

. . . .

While I am thankful for all the blind luck, blessings and good fortune that I've enjoyed throughout my life, owing to my humble origins I've never thought of myself as privileged. I realized then, perhaps for the first time, that I was, in fact, quite privileged. Financial wealth is a wonderful thing if you can get it, but most would agree that a much greater blessing is the loyalty, if not the love, of another fellow human being. When that love is manifest as a concern for your health and is shown daily in any number of small gestures that assist you on your journey toward wellness, it feels as though the Hope diamond, the Mona Lisa, and all the stars in the heavens belong to you.

We all need a little help from our friends and loved ones, but sometimes that help is not forthcoming. Before we delve into strategies for handling those situations where you find yourself alone in your efforts, let us first look at the best-case scenario when you have someone supporting you.

There are a number of popular sayings that get at the heart of what it is to be supported by someone: "Two heads are better than one" and "Many hands make light work," are just two of many. When my wife and I were doing our initial research on nutrition, we were able to split the work and cover twice as much ground in a short period of time. When it came to exercise, we encouraged each other and, in the first two months when I was still gathering information and grumbling because I hadn't lost the weight I had hoped, she comforted me. I've told her more than once that I don't think I could have made it without her, but at the risk of sounding ungrateful, and maybe even a little arrogant, I know I could have. I believe the same is true for her. Yes, it might have taken each of us a little longer had we gone about this separately, but I believe the strength of the research we did, as well as the raw power of the food we ate, would have ensured our success separately or together.

If you have the support of a friend or family member, coordinate your efforts while eliminating duplication of effort. While one of you researches foods, the other can look into the best exercise routines and equipment. Congratulate each other on your victories, no matter how small, and encourage each other when success stalls, as it inevitably will. Most important, be honest with each other. This won't always be easy. When Mary and I first walked the one-mile loop around our neighborhood, our conversations sometimes made us sad and even angry. Without realizing it, we engaged in a year and a half is worth of intensive therapy, walking in circles in the dark and pouring out our souls to each other. Not even the most committed professional counselor will get up at 4:30 am and listen to you go on about yourself the way a good friend or a spouse will. If you have such a person in your life, count yourself among the richest people you know.

Sometimes having more than one person in a household can work against you, especially when one or more members don't share your enthusiasm for better nutrition and fitness. In the case of children, I'm in favor of a governmental model akin to a benign dictatorship. I believe democracy is fine, up to a point, but if children were mature enough to make all their own decisions, technically they wouldn't be children anymore. As parents, my wife and I knew we were failing our children nutritionally. It took years for us to change, but change we did, and once we did, we insisted on the same approach to food for our children.

Because we've been there, it doesn't surprise us so much when we hear parents, in some cases degreed professionals, lament that they simply have to buy certain foods, usually junk food, for the kids because they won't eat anything else. Just like we used to, they buy substandard, high-calorie, low-nutrient foods for their kids, even though they know these foods will ultimately have a negative impact on their children's health, perhaps for the rest of their lives. I've sat in the lobby of the movie house waiting for the theatre to empty for the next showing, and watched parents buy their children "diabetes starter kits," gaily colored packages of sticky soda, stale popcorn loaded with rancid smelling soy oil and artificial butter flavoring, trans fat-laden chips, gooey, tooth rotting, mood-altering candy, all with enough monosodium glutamate, additives and preservatives to choke a horse.

For years, out of ignorance and because of our own addiction to junk food, my wife and I were guilty of the same conduct, but no more. On the rare occasion when we go to the movies with our children, we bring our own popcorn flavored with real butter. We bring raisins as well as crispy nuts. We also bring cheese, fresh or dried apples, home made beef jerky, or home made cookies. More often, we rent a movie and watch it at home. It's even easier that way to have delicious healthful snacks that we can enjoy while watching the movie.

I believe that it is the parents' poor diet and lifestyle that leaves them so fragile and vulnerable, so much so that they are willing to sacrifice their children's health by buying them what I call "shut up" food, just so they can have a little peace and quiet. The good news is that it is never too late to change. Mary and I found that when we improved our diet, we were less irritable and had a lot more patience. We found we were better able to put up with the sometimes difficult behavior of our children—and of each other. Our children have bounced back wonderfully, and so did we.

When your spouse doesn't share your enthusiasm for healthy eating, finding solutions can be more difficult. In situations like these, improving your nutrition is easier to do on your own. This isn't a practical solution when you're living under the same roof with someone else, so a compromise must be arranged. Even in the best of situations where there is agreement on most issues of nutrition and exercise, there will always still be some differences. People have to learn to negotiate these differences. For a while, I had a difficult time controlling my consumption of nuts and would eat them by the handfuls. It takes a couple of days to prepare crispy nuts, so we didn't make them all the time. I was OK as long as they weren't around, but whenever they were, I just couldn't help myself. I would have been happy if we never made them, but the rest of the family enjoyed them, too and since nuts are a very nutritious food, I had to find a solution that worked for all of us.

The compromise we reached was that Mary continued to make them, but they were hidden somewhere in the house where I couldn't see them. As long as they were out of my sight, they were out of my mind and my mouth. This arrangement worked out wonderfully until, mysteriously, I got over my "addiction" to them and was able to eat them without splurging.

These kinds of arrangements require what I call the three "C's," which are a willingness to Cooperate and Compromise Creatively. Our dilemma with the nuts proves that when you're creative, it is possible to find solutions that enable everyone to win.

In our experience, we've observed that women seem to be more willing to take the steps required to improve their health and nutrition than their husbands. Mary is often asked how she was able to get me to a point where I was willing to make a real change. The fact is that we came to the decision independently at about the same time, but there were many ways that Mary helped me after our initial decision which might be worth sharing for those of you with "difficult" spouses.

Helping your husband to get motivated

Despite our tough exteriors, men are vulnerable, too, and need as much emotional, spiritual and logistical support as any woman. One of the burdens that society places on men is that we are taught from a very young age that we should never appear to be weak or in need of help. Subsequently, we're often reluctant to ask for help. Sometimes, if help is offered in the wrong way—in the form of accusations, threats or in a tone tainted with pity—it may make us feel weak, resulting in a response that is defensive or even hostile. For a long time, Mary ignored my obesity as completely as my doctors did. She knew I was sensitive to the issue and didn't know how to address it without hurting my feelings. The solution was to approach the issue in a manner that I was more receptive to. I happen to be a very goal-oriented person who likes to apply logic and reason to solve problems.

Chapter Sixteen: Ten Steps To A New Life

Mary eventually came to understand this and broached my weight problem as if it were any other mechanical problem that had a logical solution. She engaged her medical background and focused on the physiological underpinnings of obesity. The human body is, in many ways like a machine, just infinitely more complex. By addressing the problem this way, without any fuzzy emotional baggage, I was much more motivated toward finding a solution, because like most men, I tend to view solutions as a product of logic and reason, rather than emotion. From this starting point, I could then delve into the deeper, and sometimes more painful, emotional reasons that contributed to my health problems.

Mary was a real partner in my effort to change my behavior and reclaim my health. She never made me feel guilty when I felt like giving up. When I accused her of not being there for me, she did not respond with bitterness as she might have in the past, but instead replied with composure and the kind of reason that I had no choice but to respect. By treating me in this manner, she made it easier for me to treat her in kind. I was finally able to resist the urge I always had to solve her problems for her—in five minutes or less—and could turn off my analytical mind and just listen to what she had to say. I found that more often than not, she already had her solution and just wanted me to listen and perhaps share the burden of shouldering a difficult decision.

One of the most powerful motivators that Mary employed that helped me be successful was cooking. For a long time, there was very little cooking that went on in our house. More often than not, we frequented restaurants, ate take-out food, ordered pizza, or thawed and reheated pre-cooked frozen foods. When Mary did cook, it was often done with such careless execution that the dish itself became a gustatory proclamation of her disdain for cooking.

For example, if we were short a few ingredients for a dish, she would make it anyway, without any concern for the quality of the end product. Once she substituted parsley for cilantro in my favorite salsa recipe, because, as she explained, "they're both green." On another occasion, she discovered a recipe for goulash which included among its principal ingredients frozen vegetables, ground beef and barbecue sauce. Since the only ingredient that had to be cooked was the meat, it was an easy dish to make. As it turned out, it was too easy. She served it for nearly two weeks in a row until the entire family threatened to run away from home.

Once she began to discover real food and real cooking, our home and our palates were transformed. After work, I was no longer tempted to pull into a fast food drive-thru to get something to eat before going home to dinner. Each new day brought with it the tantalizing tastes and smells of real food cooked from scratch. I started calling home an hour or so before 5:00 pm to inquire about the evening's meal, like a kid asking Santa Claus for a sneak peak at his gift list. It wasn't just the fact that the food was delicious it was also doing me a lot of good. In a very short span of time, I noticed that I felt better, my clothes fit better, I was stronger, and the aches and pains that I woke up with every morning were disappearing. Mary was changing, too. She smiled more often and seemed more alive than even before we were married 16 years earlier. My oldest daughter, who had been steadily gaining weight, was now losing weight, and my youngest, who suffered from frightful mood swings, had transformed into a little angel.

Even though she was the full-time manager of our home, Mary somehow found the time to cook as well. It sounds impossible, I know, but she was able to do all this because the food changed her as much as it changed me. She was stronger, happier and, for the first time in her life, free of the depression that had clouded her path for so many years.

Likewise, I, too took my turn in the kitchen and found that the only thing more enjoyable than eating a wonderful meal is preparing one for the people you love.

Step 4: Create harmony in your life

If you've ever been to a concert and listened to the orchestra warm up, you know just how disconcerting that cacophony of sound can be.

Chapter Sixteen: Ten Steps To A New Life

Imagine trying to concentrate on something important with that noise going on in your ear. Now imagine how difficult it can be to develop healthier habits for someone distracted by the "noise" of out-of-control debt, a bad relationship or career problems.

The idea that you can make positive change in one part of your life while the rest of your life is a complete disaster is nonsense. It may be temporarily possible for someone with extreme willpower, but for most of us, the greater the sum of all our troubles combined, the more difficult it is to resolve any one of those troubles. Have you ever wondered why, after breaking up with someone you've been close to, that person can seem more appealing and attractive than ever? This is due to our natural inclination to desire the things that are least attainable, but it is also due to the fact that once the stress of a bad relationship has been removed, people find they are able to get back to living again.

Perhaps the problem is not a relationship, but debt and financial problems that are impeding your health goals. In a worst case scenario, where debt collectors are stalking you at home and at the office, the stress can wear you down and drive you to indulge in the kind of food and nonproductive behavior that will only make your health problems worse. The solution is to take stock of your life and make an honest list of the things you want to change. Prioritize that list, then attack each item on that list in turn. Mounting debt and unfulfilling careers were two of the stresses that contributed to our poor health. But we created a plan, paid off our debts and changed our careers. With that weight lifted from our shoulders, getting the weight off our middles was considerably easier.

Your life is an orchestra. To realize the beautiful music that you're capable of living, you've got to get each section—the percussion, wind instruments and the strings, your debts, relationships and career sections—playing the same song.

Step 5: Simplify your life

My oldest daughter played soccer in a junior league for a time when she was younger. At one of the games once, Mary met a woman who seemed to be on the verge of a nervous breakdown and wasn't enjoying the game at all. Her daughter played soccer, but she also had a son who was playing on another soccer team, at the same time, some distance away. The poor woman had been driving back and forth between games so that she could be in attendance for both children.

I've known quite a few parents with children enrolled in a number of extra curricular activities. Besides the chauffeuring, team practices, and related expenses, these parents have jobs, and in some cases, attend church services and other regular appointments—orthodontists, pediatricians, allergy specialists, psychiatrists, learning specialists—two or three times a week. When your life is this crazy, it is impossible to cook, exercise and get enough sleep. The solution to this dilemma is not to ask, "How do I manage my crazy life?" but to apply the Socratic method and ask, "Do I need this crazy life?" Very often the answer is "no" because what children want most from their parents is not horseback riding lessons, but their time and attention. Enriching your child's life is a wonderful goal, but it should not be done at the expense of your sanity.

In 2004, we turned off our television set for good. My frustration with television had been building since the decline in availability of free, over-the-air reception and the steady rise in cable fees. I was offended by the mindless vulgarity of the programming—and that was just the children's shows—and the endless messages telling me that I and my family were less worthy if we didn't spend all our money on the paycheck-absorbing products and services frequently advertised.

In George Orwell's novel, *1984*, the principal character lives in a world governed by an oppressive regime where "telescreens," two-way televisions, are installed in every home. These screens are monitored by "Big Brother" and provide a means for the government to broadcast the party politics to all citizens and reinforce state sanctioned "groupthink." In Orwell's world, diversity of opinion is not tolerated.

Television in the real world has a similar power to propagate groupthink and shape ideas by limiting differing opinions and alternative views. Of course, the same can be said of other traditional media: radio, newspapers and magazines, as well as the newest medium, the Internet. But television, through its ubiquity and raw visceral power to command our attention, is unlike anything else in our history.

When the cable service was finally disconnected, the peaceful sound of silence descended into our lives. Raven, the youngest member of our family and the one most susceptible to the siren song of television, began spending more of her free time reading and drawing. We also noted that her RTM (Requests for Toys per Minute) and her RFM (Requests For McDonald's) dropped significantly immediately after the screen went black. Stephanie, our oldest daughter, who somehow was born with a natural immunity to television, used what little time she had formerly allotted for TV to spend reading the work of great fiction writers. Mary used her newly found time to reconnect with out-of-state family, to cook and read, and to apply her medical background to the study of human nutrition and food metabolism.

Of all the changes wrought by our newfound freedom from TV, mine was the most astonishing. I had long complained about my lack of time and now found myself with a surplus. Suddenly there was all the time in the world to do the things I needed to do, which included focusing more on my health. In time, we canceled our mobile phone plan and purchased a pay-as-you-go mobile plan instead. It was less expensive and less hassle.

Auto retailers are the chief advertisers on TV. I had planned, for some time, to buy a new car, but without the constant drone of "buy, buy, buy" in my mind on a daily basis, I suddenly saw the superior logic of simply repairing the old car. I did not realize how much my purchasing decisions had been affected by television.

By letting go of some of the trappings of commercialism, we came to discover what was really most important. One of the most interesting and pleasant outcomes of these changes was that by ignoring the "Call of the Mall," we found ourselves with a surplus of income at the end of every month.

Step 6: Eat as if your life depended on it

The convenience and junk food sectors of the food industry and their supporters have spent billions to convince us to buy more and eat more. We have been told that it absolutely does not matter what we put into our bodies, as long as we exercise moderation and, of course, get plenty of physical exercise. Many of us have bought into this lie and many have paid a heavy price for following this advice.

One of the best ways to break out of the vicious cycle of poor nutrition and yoyo dieting is just to avoid processed foods. Another is to start cooking your own meals. In the past, this was easier said than done, but I found that eating whole foods reduced my cravings for junk, and gave me the energy and motivation to cook.

Step 7: Make exercise a part of your life

No one has to be convinced that exercise is important. The problem has always been how do you make regular exercise a habit? Exercise, like almost everything else, can only become a habit if we take some pleasure in it. I found that being on a low-energy diet left me with little ability to enjoy exercise.

The chief irony of the low-fat paradigm is in the oft-repeated advice to eat less, and at the same time, exercise more. This is not unlike advising someone to put less gas in their car, while expecting them to drive farther. This upside-down logic has been the bane of dieters for decades. My experience has led me to the following conclusions regarding exercise:

- I adopted a flexible energy-dense diet that satisfies my energy needs. When I'm going on a 5 mile hike, I know I need more energy than when I'm sitting at my desk in the office, so what I eat changes to reflect my activity.

- I built diversity into my exercise sessions. If you like running, try biking or hiking for a change of pace. Alternate between aerobic workouts and anaerobic ones like resistance training.
- If you're new to exercise, get help from a knowledgeable friend or a professional trainer. Trainers can be really affordable, and you don't need to make a lifelong commitment to them.
- I listen to my body and take time off whenever I feel like I need a rest. Don't overwork yourself. Injuries can be painful, time consuming and can even throw you off track for extended periods.
- Look for opportunities to make exercise a practical part of your life. My two-hour long walking sessions with Mary have more to do with sharing our lives and addressing business issues than they do with exercise, but it is great that we can have a business meeting and get a workout, too.

Step 8: Get high quality sleep

When my weight was in excess of 400 pounds, getting a good night's sleep was somewhere between difficult and impossible. The only position I could lie down in with a minimal amount of distress was on my back. Sleep apnea ensured that on most mornings, I awoke as tired as I was when I went to sleep. I often stayed up until the early hours of the morning, watching television or surfing the web—anything to delay having to go to bed.

Like many people, Mary and I had busy schedules, so after changing our diets, we decided that if we were going to find the time to exercise, we would have to get up earlier in the mornings. We began going to bed at 9:00 pm so that we could wake up by 4:00 am. It was actually easy to do this, because of our energizing diet. This was the beginning of what has become a two year habit for us, a habit we love.

It took a while before I made the connection between sleep and how much better I felt. I realized it wasn't just that I was getting enough sleep, but that I was sleeping on a regular schedule. Babies intuitively understand the importance of a consistent sleep schedule. Recent news stories suggest that medical researchers are beginning to understand it, too.

Step 9: Find your motivation

Besides being a worthwhile personal goal, improving your health is an empowering experience. If this was my only goal, however, I think I would get bored very quickly. Being healthy for the sake of being healthy just isn't enough sometimes. As a species, humans are engineered to test themselves against the world they live in and seek those goals that seem unreachable. I guess this is why some men climb mountains and why some women fly into space.

Your goals provide the motivation that helps you maintain your commitment. Without goals, the desire to push on when you feel like quitting is diminished. Figure out what you want to do with your life. Don't be shy. You can start a business, get an education, or work up the nerve to introduce yourself to the man or woman you want to spend the rest of your life with. Whatever your goals are, recognize them, name them, and start planning to achieve them.

Step 10: Share what you've learned

Half the fun of learning how to live a life full of passion is in helping others to do the same. When the time comes, share what you know, and ask that your only compensation be that they do the same for someone else, when they are ready.

Chapter Seventeen

Some Frequently Asked Questions

I'm glad you asked that

The following is a short list of questions that come up regularly. The answers cover some of the important things we learned in our efforts to improve our knowledge about food, weight loss and nutrition.

Question: What are your credentials?

Answer: I have more than ten years' experience under my belt, figuratively and literally, as a fat man. For almost 30 years I was an unwilling participant in one of the longest running medical trials to date: the Low-Fat Lifestyle trial, which began somewhere around the mid-seventies and is still going strong today. I also participated in the High Fructose Corn Syrup trial, which began at about the same time.

I've been in the trenches. I've seen the disastrous results of our failed nutrition policy from the inside. I've lost friends and family members to this policy. The suggestion behind the "credentials" question is "How dare you presume to challenge the status quo of medical orthodoxy?" I dare indeed, and so should anyone else who has found nothing but failure in the policy we now have.

Anyone who can read is free to learn as much as they want. Access to knowledge and the ability to form our own opinions is a right guaranteed to all citizens. I cannot think of a more appropriate application of those immortal words, "Life, liberty and the pursuit of happiness," than to the pursuit of better health.

Question: I've heard it said that there are no good or bad foods, just poor choices. Isn't that right?

Answer: Some health experts are very fond of this idea. They rationalize that any food can be part of a healthy diet. When they talk about poor choices, they're referring more to the quantity of the foods you consume, not so much to the quality. The injury wrought by certain foods will vary across a population group based on the relative fitness of each individual. Thus, a small child whose body has yet to be ravaged by decades of poor eating might have a higher tolerance for soda than his father, a 45-year-old Type 2 diabetic. Does this mean that it's OK for the child to take up soda as a lifelong habit, perhaps with the possibility of becoming a diabetic like his dad or should he eschew soda altogether in favor of a more healthful beverage, like raw milk? Many experts are loath to come right out and say that some foods are worthless and that we do ourselves more harm than good by consuming them, even in moderation.

When I was honest with myself, I realized there were certain foods that were absolutely bad for me in the following ways:

1. Eating even a moderate amount of these foods made me want more, and kept my cravings at a high level.

2. They were high-calorie low-nutrient foods that exerted a cumulatively negative load on my body. Refined sugar was the worst.

3. Even a small portion of some foods had an immediate and negative impact on my health. Ultra-pasteurized milk made me violently ill, and MSG gave me headaches.

4. They negatively affected me emotionally. Sugar substitutes and a vegetarian diet left me irritable and ill-tempered.

5. They satisfied my taste, but not my need. Soy products can be engineered to taste approximately like real food, but they always left me unsatisfied and fueled my desire to eat more.

6. They were killing me.

I realized that it only made sense to eliminate these foods from my diet, as they were part of the problem. No one would suggest that an alcoholic learn to drink in moderation. Why do we sabotage people with poor nutrition by encouraging them to continue eating the very foods that are at the root of their problem? In truth, the only true beneficiaries of this myth are food manufacturers and retailers.

Question: Whole foods sound good, but I could never live without my favorite foods. How did you do it?

Answer: I don't live without my favorite foods because I eat all the foods I want to eat. The most difficult thing for me to grasp initially was the fact that my tastes and preferences would change. I did not think I could ever live without commercial potato chips, but now I no longer crave them.

I think it's because the food I eat satisfies me completely. I no longer want or need any of the processed junk I used to eat. As for favorite comfort foods, I like ice cream, ginger ale, pizza and even candy now and then. I eat all of these things. The difference is that they're all homemade, they contain no additives. And because the foods I eat are satisfying, I can eat them in moderation.

Question: Isn't it wrong to deprive yourself of your favorite foods?

Answer: Food industry propagandists and their supporters in the medical field are quite fond of the don't-deprive-yourself-or-you'll-develop-an-obsession school of thought. They even have the studies to prove it. I find it interesting that no one believes that depriving yourself of bashing your neighbor on the head, no matter how much you might want to, will somehow lead to a career as a mugger. And yet, there is this belief that not letting your children drink soda today will cause them to uncontrollably swill gallons of the stuff when they're older.

The problem is that people really don't understand the nature of deprivation. Simply put, you cannot be deprived of something you do not desire. I found low-fat fake food diets to be all about deprivation, because they kept me in a constant state of desire for something more fulfilling. Once I switched to a balanced diet of whole foods, I was satisfied. Once I was satisfied, my desire for processed foods ceased. No desire, no deprivation.

Question: I saw a study that proved you could lose weight eating nothing but convenience food. Doesn't that invalidate your argument about convenience foods?

Answer: I'm not surprised. If you look hard enough, you can find a study that supports any hypothesis you can come up with. This is because studies can be easily engineered to produce any results you want. Many studies are funded by parties with a vested interest in a positive outcome. Most people would call this a conflict of interest, but in the strange and curious world of medical research, this is called business as usual. Unscrupulous researchers can make a study "dance" in a number of ways. I'll list just a few here:

- If you're testing a drug that will be administered to sick people, give it to the healthiest "sick" people you can find and give the placebo to the sickest sick people you can find to ensure that the study results will be positive.
- If the results of the study at 12-months are disastrous, pretend the study was for only six months and report those results instead.
- Obscure the results of a study by focusing on relative risk (which makes the differences seem large) while downplaying the absolute risks. In other words, report study results in

percentages rather than absolute numbers. For example, if Joe hits Larry two times with a cricket bat before being dosed with a new anti-aggression drug, but only hits Larry one time after being dosed, we can report a 50 percent reduction in aggressive behavior—an impressive dose response indeed. Never mind, that we're only talking about two data points. Further, if Joe falls over from a heart attack due to an unintended side effect of the drug, simply bury that small fact somewhere in the study as a "statistically insignificant event."

- Lie.

Question: Doesn't eating better quality food cost more?

Answer: Yes, if you look only at the amount you pay at the checkout counter. Too often we focus on the near-term cost of food while ignoring the long-term consequences. A lifetime of eating nutrient-poor foods along with cheap, low-fat dairy and egg substitutes sapped the strength from both my body and my wallet.

Over the long term, I paid a high price for junk food in prescription and over the counter medicines, missed days from work, and a diminished quality of life.

Question: Isn't weight management simply a matter of calories in/calories out?

Answer: If it was that simple, losing weight would be easy. Just cut back on the number of calories consumed, and you'll magically lose weight. Of course, most experienced dieters know that losing weight is anything but simple. In the real world, when you cut back on calories, you get hungry. When you remain in this state for an extended period, you're more likely to binge eat. Cutting back too much on calories can trigger a "starvation" signal to the body to conserve energy (fat), so you can't lose weight no matter how little you eat.

Much of the advice regarding proper nutrition for maintaining an appropriate weight is based on quantity. Sure, we're told we can eat all the vegetables we want, but for everything else, we are advised to manage the amount and balance that against what we expend in exercise.

The problem with this advice is that it is woefully simplified and thus unusable for many people. In my case, it simply did not work for me. First, few of us know how many calories we actually expend walking up a flight of stairs, watching TV or running five miles. If we don't know how many calories we're burning, how can we possibly know how many calories to consume? Second, the calories in/calories out equation ignores the importance of food quality while overemphasizing food quantity. Eating low-quality foods can work against your efforts to be healthy. In my case, they prevented me from losing weight successfully.

What I eventually discovered was that the type of food I ate could trigger weight loss or weight gain. I learned that some foods affected me emotionally, making me irritable, while other foods left me so fatigued that I was often too tired to exercise. Finally, I discovered that my body really didn't like the idea of losing weight and would adapt to increased exercise with an increase in energy conservation. This is why the same amount and type of exercise that worked for me at first stopped working for me six months later. Why health experts continue to ignore many of these complicating factors of the calories in/calories out equation remains a mystery to me, even today.

Question: I heard that for weight loss, a balanced diet should consist of about 55 to 60 percent carbohydrates, and be low in fat. Is this a good strategy for losing weight and staying healthy?

Answer: I found this to be true only if my dieting strategy was to get really, really, fat. I grew up in the era of the four food groups, later replaced by the food pyramid. Carbohydrates are prominently positioned in the pyramid, sending the message that we should eat more of them, so I was shocked when I discovered that livestock producers place pigs and cows on high carbohydrate diets to fatten them up. Conversely, increasing the percentage of the right kind of fat in my diet resulted in a

. . . .

corresponding decrease in body weight. No one ever told me that carbohydrates, along with protein, can be converted into stored body fat. The message that all dietary fat equals body fat was a lie that I believed for years—even after I cut fat consumption drastically—and continued to gain weight.

In truth, such a diet might work for helping some people to lose weight, but if you've been following this advice and it hasn't worked for you, it might be wise to consider other alternatives. Additionally, separate from the issue of losing weight, we have to consider whether a high plant-based processed foods diet is healthy. When you consider the relentless increase of heart disease and cancer in this country, it certainly gives reason to pause and ask whether diet is not a contributing factor.

Question: Aren't fruit juices a healthy alternative to sodas?

Answer: Fruits contain a simple sugar called fructose. For a time, I actually believed that fruit juice was a diet drink, dutifully consuming large quantities of juice after exercising. Even though the juices were very sweet, I didn't think of them as a source of "sugar." Sugar was a white granular substance that came in a bag or a box from the grocery store. Fruit juice was "natural," I reasoned. I believed that as long as I was careful about my consumption of white sugar, I could drink fruit juice to my heart's content. I had no idea how much sugar I was consuming in the form of juices, as well as just about every convenience food product I purchased, since most of them contain some form of added sugar, often in the form of high fructose corn syrup. Because the dietary experts spent so much time emphasizing dietary fat as the source of my obesity, I ignored the mountains of sugar that were hidden in everything I consumed, from tomato sauce to "healthy" cereals.

Question: Eating fat makes you fat, right?

Answer: Maybe so, maybe not. Our bodies use glucose for energy. Most of that energy comes in the form of sugars and starches from plant sources such as fruits, vegetables and grains. Milk is a notable exception as a source of sugar in that it has lactose (milk sugar), but comes from an animal source. What is less well known is that our bodies can utilize fat as an energy source as well.

I found that when I was consuming dietary fat along with sugar, starches, and grains, which comprised the bulk of my diet, I gained weight. Like most people, I assumed it was the fat in my diet that was making me fat. When I transitioned to a more balanced, traditional foods diet that reduced the amounts of sugar, starch, grains, along with most processed foods, I could eat fat and still lose weight.

Question: What's wrong with asking my doctor about how to lose weight?

Answer: Nothing, if your doctor is educated in the complexities of nutrition and weight loss. I've had several doctors over the years, and they were all great people, but none of them, not one, could give me any useful advice about weight loss.

The family doctor is great when it comes to the "simple" things, like broken bones, diagnosing an illness based on a predefined list of symptoms, administering physicals and writing prescriptions. They are trained to recognize and deal with acute disease issues and other obvious abnormalities. We would all fare poorly without them, but when it comes to long term chronic conditions, like obesity, the slow killer, they are less skilled and tend to rely on useless advice, such as advising you to "just stop eating so much."

Simply knowing that a diet high in refined carbohydrates can cause weight gain while reducing carbs and adding good fats can help some people lose weight goes a long way toward providing obese people with basic advice that they can actually use. This isn't fringe science; any decent 101 level anatomy and physiology textbook lays out the basics of macronutrient metabolism, but until the recent attention on how carbohydrates and fats are metabolized in the body, most doctors would have told you the opposite. Many still will.

Chapter Seventeen: Some Frequently Asked Questions

. . . .

The fact that there are doctors with weight problems of their own highlights the difficulties involved in losing weight. I believe the ideal doctor-patient relationship exists when both parties utilize their strengths to help each other. Patients should make an honest effort to tell the truth about their condition instead of simply accepting a treatment plan that they know will fail. Doctors should unburden themselves of the pressure to have all the answers, recognize the limits of their knowledge, and partner with their patients to find workable solutions.

Question: None of this really applies to me since I'm thin, right?

Answer: There's an old saying that says you can never be too rich, too thin or too beautiful. While I agree with the first and last items, I take issue with the second. While it's possible to be thin and healthy, the idea that being thin always equals health is a myth perpetuated by popular culture and the fashion and entertainment industries. I'm no exception to this disease of the mind. I, too, wanted to be thin and assumed that low body weight directly correlated with good health.

When I was a vegetarian, I lost fifty pounds and certainly looked healthier than I once did, but I knew that inside it was a different story. I was weak and lacked the strength I once had. I had headaches, was irritable, lacked focus, had digestion problems and generally felt bad on most days. I ate lots of fruits and vegetables, kept dietary fat to a minimum, ate soy everyday and didn't drink or smoke, and yet, I felt awful.

The fallacy of thin is having a tragic effect on a generation of young women who try desperately to emulate the emaciated females they see in the popular media. These misguided women drift through their daily lives gaunt and hollow-eyed, with sunken cheeks and pallid skin in a perpetual state of nutrient starvation. Someone needs to tell these waifs that there's nothing sexy about starvation. Their appearance only tells half the story. The rest—what is happening to their bodies on the inside— does not become apparent until later.

Chapter Eighteen

Rebirth
The end is just the beginning

It has been over two years since Mary and I began our journey. We could not have foreseen what was to come of the simple idea to change what we ate.

One of the wonderful results of my transformation is this book. I have always loved to write, but for years lacked the courage to take that first step. I thank you, the reader, for making the effort worthwhile by sharing with me a portion of your time. Along with other titles in the works, I've taken my story, and my message to the streets in the hopes that those people who once thought the course of their lives predetermined can see that it is possible to change and do it on their own terms. As a former teacher, there's nothing I enjoy more than talking to people and encouraging them to visualize a better future for themselves.

Cleaning up my diet cleaned up my body, my mind and my life. I am able to think more clearly now and see opportunities that I could never have seen before because I was too wrapped up in the physical and emotional problems created and exacerbated by poor health.

My education in the value of traditional foods continues at a brisk pace, as do my efforts toward self-improvement. Physically, I am free of the aches and pains, sleep apnea, asthma, mild depression and hypertension that once plagued me.

A Life Unburdened

We are big supporters of independent food producers and purchase much of our food from local farmers. The return on our investment, in health, has been nothing short of a miracle. Conversely, our investment in over the counter and prescription medicines has been reduced to zero. In fact, it has been two years since I last caught a cold. I'm sharper mentally and my personal zeal for life burns brighter now than it has in years. Mary, thankfully free of medication as well, has had a similar experience. We still arise at 4:00 am several times a week to take our two-hour walk where we talk in the quiet hours before sunrise. Each new day for us is a special blessing that we cherish as if it is our last.

Our daughters have experienced a miraculous change as well. They exercise regularly, and are considerably more fit than they once were. They know how to read product labels and how to critically evaluate ubiquitous and often dubious food health claims. They rarely fall ill now and when they do feel out of sorts, a good night's rest has always solved the problem. We're teaching them how to cook and we lead by example by making sure we always eat breakfast and sit down together as a family for the evening meal.

It's hard to believe that less than three years ago I thought my life was over. I find it impossible to convey just how thankful I am for this second chance.

On a walk with my oldest daughter one morning, I asked her what she thought of the many changes her mother and I have made and the challenges we've faced as a family. She thought for a moment and replied, "We're happier now."

She was right.

RESOURCES

- *The Second Brain : A Groundbreaking New Understanding of Nervous Disorders of the Stomach and Intestine* — by Michael Gershon
- *Nourishing Traditions: The Cookbook that Challenges Politically Correct Nutrition and the Diet Dictocrats* — by Sally Fallon, Mary G. Enig, PhD.
- *Safe Food: Bacteria, Biotechnology, and Bioterrorism* — by Marion Nestle
- *Food Politics: How the Food Industry Influences Nutrition and Health* — by Marion Nestle
- *Fast Food Nation: The Dark Side of the All-American Meal* — by Eric Schlosser
- *Fat Land : How Americans Became the Fattest People in the World* — by Greg Critser
- *The Cholesterol Myths : Exposing the Fallacy that Saturated Fat and Cholesterol Cause Heart Disease* — by Uffe Ravnskov
- *Know Your Fats : The Complete Primer for Understanding the Nutrition of Fats, Oils and Cholesterol* — by Mary G. Enig, PhD.
- *The Hungry Gene: The Inside Story of the Obesity Industry* — Ellen Ruppel Shell
- *Eat Fat, Lose Fat:* — Dr. Mary Enig, PhD. and Sally Fallon
- *A Consumer's Dictionary of Food Additives* – Ruth Winter. M.S.
- *The Whole Soy Story: The dark side of America's favorite health food* – Kaayla T. Daniel, PhD, CCN
- *"The Soft Science of Dietary Fat,"* Journal Science (March 30, 2001, Volume 291, pages 2536-2545) http://www.sciencemag.org
- The Weston A. Price Foundation http://www.westonaprice.org
- The Omnivore http://www.theomnivore.com
- The International Network of Cholesterol Skeptics: http://www.thincs.org

Richard Morris is a writer, publisher, real food activist, health researcher, speaker and self-described nutrition contrarian. An ardent supporter of fair trade for the family farm, Richard is the creator and chief instigator at BreadandMoney.com, a web site that extolls the virtues of traditional foods and suburban homesteading.

To arrange a speaking engagement with your group or to provide feedback on this book, you can reach Richard at this address: feedback@breadandmoney.com or write to the publisher at Miralibri Press / P.O. Box 2452 Woodbridge, VA 22195